The Nurse and the Dying Patient

The Nurse
and the
Dying Patient

RT
86
.Q5

Jeanne C. Quint, M. S., R. N.

**Assistant Research Sociologist, School of Nursing
University of California, San Francisco**

*The Macmillan Company, New York
Collier-Macmillan Publishers, London*

The Macmillan Company
866 Third Avenue, New York, New York 10022

Collier-Macmillan Canada, Ltd., Toronto, Ontario

Library of Congress catalog card number: 67-14418

Printing: 1 2 3 4 5 6 7 8   Year: 3 4 5 6 7 8 9

NOT THE DYING

Thus, too Admetus found it,
long ago, when his Alcestis
took the dying from him and
gave back a greater terror,
death. It's not the dying
stills the heart within us.
Death comes not to the dying
or the dead, but to
the living, from whose heart
it draws its life—until the dying
comes in mercy and
takes back this death.

WAYNE DODD
American Scholar, Summer, 1965

Foreword

The first schools of nursing in the United States were established almost 100 years ago. Since that time thousands of nurse students and graduates have been faced with problems associated with care and comfort of dying patients and with support of families under the stresses occasioned by long-impending or sudden death of a family member. Miss Quint's timely book brings to the reader both a sense of shock and a sense of revelation. The sense of shock comes from the sudden realization that so little attention has been given in years past to preparing nurses to cope effectively with problems associated with dying. The sense of revelation comes from the equally sudden realization that so much can be done, not only to enable nurses to provide the care and comfort that is so much needed by patients and their families during periods of extreme stress, but also to achieve the sense of personal worthwhileness and fulfillment which comes from the knowledge of work well done.

Miss Quint's book is a part of a larger study carried on at the University of California School of Nursing, San Francisco Medical Center, of how nursing and medical personnel give care to dying patients. Data for Miss Quint's study were obtained primarily through unstructured interviews with students and teachers in five schools of nursing in the San Francisco Bay area, one of which was a university school and four of which were hospital schools. In the university school, interviews were held with students enrolled in registered nurse baccalaureate and graduate programs in nursing, as well as with those enrolled in the basic baccalaureate program.

The theme of Miss Quint's book may be stated as follows: "The dying patient's behavior is a function of his interactions with significant persons around him. If these interactions are such that the patient is enabled to live each moment as it comes, he will gain the added psychological strength he needs to face the approach of death."

In discussing questions of how nurse students can be prepared to cope effectively with difficult nursing problems associated with care of dying patients, Miss Quint identifies problem areas which should be of great concern to both schools of nursing and nursing service agencies and to physicians and nurses. These include the lack of a common agreement as to "what is good" in relation to patient care and the lack of awareness of what may happen to both students and patients in the highly complex situations in which care is being provided. Miss Quint discusses the difficult problems which arise when nurse teachers are unsure of how to teach and unprepared for reactions of students. She emphasizes the facts that students may be faced with what to them are overwhelming assignments and that, in attempting to cope with the assignments, they may fail to live up to their own unrealistic expectations of themselves. She suggests that nurse students need to be held accountable for what they say as well as what they do, but that effective teaching in relation to verbal communication cannot take place unless there is cooperation between teachers and ward nurses and consistency in their concepts of what constitutes good nursing practice.

Not only are problems of basic students discussed, but also those of registered nurses who, when they return to school, are faced with the impact of a system which attempts to alter their previously established patterns of working with patients. When nurses who have seen themselves as competent and effective are suddenly confronted with the general directive to provide psychological support to critically ill patients and their families, the requirement that they learn new ways of functioning may, at least for a time, threaten their own sense of security. With these nurses, too, the roles of nurse teachers and the nurse practitioners are crucial.

In Chapter 8 Miss Quint makes concrete proposals for changes in nursing programs to facilitate better care for dying patients and more satisfying experiences for nurses. These include the need for a planned and coordinated teaching program during the first year centered specifically on nursing care of dying patients—assignments through which students will be enabled to confront their feelings rather than push them aside; assistance of sensitive, perceptive nurse teachers who are knowledgeable about human behavior and what happens to patients in hospitals; better communication between nurse teachers and nursing service personnel and between nurses and physicians about care of individual patients; involvement of the medical staff in cooperative planning for better services to dying patients; and provision for guidance and support on a regular basis to nursing staff involved in care. In planning a teaching program she emphasizes the need to enable students to understand the philosophic and pragmatic issues associated with dying, as well as the cultural patterns and societal values. She believes that initial and later explorations at the intellectual level help to prepare students for concrete realities. She discusses the past and current emphasis in the health professions on life saving as a primary occupational value and the impact of this on the care that dying patients receive. She feels that innovations in teaching and practice of nursing are needed, including the ability to break old, established patterns of dealing with physicians and the courage to intercede in behalf of patients. She states that a new philosophy of nursing practice is needed which emphasizes that patients' rights and nurses' responsibilities involve more than simple carrying out of doctor orders. She concludes that the "dying patient— the forgotten man in the hospital—can well use an ally whose goal it is to help him with his human problems; that the professional nurse can assume this function if she is willing to accept the risks of moving into new kinds of role relationships with physicians, patients, families, and all manner of professional and nonprofessional personnel."

The task of preparing such nurses is the task of the nursing school. Meeting the task may well require revolutionary changes in curriculum planning and implementation, teacher preparation, relationships between education and service personnel and between physicians and nurses, and in concepts of nursing care and the role of the nurse. For the thousands of patients for whom nurses will care in the years to come and for the welfare of the nurses themselves, the stakes are very high. Nursing schools have been confronted with the need for change in years past, and have faced up to the problems that change involves. As new research findings become available they will undoubtedly meet the challenge of continued change. In so doing, not only will the professional role of the nurse continue to evolve, but also the role of nursing as an irreplaceable component of the health care spectrum.

HELEN NAHM
Dean, School of Nursing
University of California
San Francisco

Preface

From the relative protection of middle-class American life, young women who enter schools of nursing abruptly find themselves immersed in a world in which many basic values and personal beliefs are tested and often threatened. They have chosen an occupation which brings them face to face with many of the sorrows of human existence—suffering and pain, illness and crippling, and death. The transition to nursing brings the students into contact with many emotionally disturbing events and activities. Yet nursing curricula have not been organized to provide them with systematic help in coping with the emotional distress and personal conflict associated with many of these experiences. This book reports on what happens to students of nursing during and after their encounters with one stress-producing problem—death—but the reader should be aware that these students encounter many other identity stresses in the course of learning to be nurses.

The book is one in a series resulting from a six-year investigation supported by Public Health Service Research Grant No. NU00047 from the Division of Nursing, Bureau of State Services–Community Health. Directed by Anselm L. Strauss, the project was conducted at the School of Nursing, University of California Medical Center, San Francisco, California. The members of the research team were Jeanne C. Quint and Barney G. Glaser. Reflecting a sociological perspective, the study as a whole was focused upon what happens to hospital staff and to patients during the process of death. A first monograph describing interactional patterns involving the patients, their families, and the hospital staff was published in 1965 under the title *Awareness of Dying*. This second book describes how nursing students learn about death as an occupational problem. The data were provided by five schools of nursing in the San Francisco area.

In the United States, death is an unpopular idea. Increasingly, persons who are dying are being segregated from the rest of society—usually in hospitals and convalescent homes. At the same time, modern medical technology is producing many devices capable of prolonging life. In consequence of these two facts, members of the healing professions are today facing many serious and difficult problems in providing care for dying patients in hospitals. There are several reasons why dying patients pose special problems for nurses. Because the ending of human life is a critical experience of separation in this society, the dying patient and his family are often emotionally upset. Like other Americans, many nurses are not particularly comfortable in the presence of a person who is dying, nor can they converse easily with him about his forthcoming death. Although physicians have definite responsibilities for and must make specific decisions about dying patients, within the hospital nurses must deal with the day-by-day interactions with these patients and their families. Conversations with dying patients and their families are commonplace in nursing practice, yet nurses avoid many of these conversations in much the same way as do laymen.

As students, nurses have been taught how to take care of the dying patient's body. They have had little specialized preparation for dealing with the many interactional problems which take place when a patient is dying. As the reader will become aware, educational programs in nursing reflect the values, beliefs, and practices of the wider society in which they emerge. The general taboo about death has resulted in nursing curricula which have given minimal attention to many serious issues and difficult decisions which nurses face in providing care for dying patients and their families. Phrased somewhat differently, cultural values concerning death have led to a gap in the education of nurses and, in turn, to a gap in the nursing services available to patients who are dying. Undoubtedly the curricula in medical schools show a similar gap.

Any occupational group providing direct services to individuals in need must sometimes provide services which are not easy to provide. For nurses, providing care for dying patients is one such service, but death is only one of many stress-producing problems which nurses meet in practice. One can assume that teachers in public schools, social workers, lawyers, physicians, policemen, and many others engaged in working with people encounter occupational problems which are personally disturbing and not easily solved or readily forgotten. Close scrutiny of the educational programs offered any of these groups would probably show a gap in the training experiences provided for work problems which cause the practitioner to experience conflict because basic values and personal beliefs are at stake. Undoubtedly the services offered to the public also suffer a deficit because the occupational problems at issue do not usually have simple yes or no solutions but rather are heavily influenced by the practitioner's value judgments. The issues raised by the findings reported in this book are neither simple nor relevant solely to the education of nurses.

I wish to thank the many people who made this book possible. I am indebted to Anselm Strauss and Barney Glaser for their support and encouragement during the many different and difficult phases of the study. I wish to thank the many persons who took time to read and comment on the original manuscript; among these were Mrs. Esther Blanc, Mrs. Shirley Chater, Fred Davis,

Mrs. Betty Dietrich, Miss Jeannette Folta, Miss Betty Highley, Miss Sally Lambert, Mrs. Mildred McIntyre, Miss Helen Nahm, Miss Katherine Rottier, and Louis Schaw. For their unique and very useful comments about the manuscript, I am especially grateful to Stewart Perry, Miss Virginia Olesen, Miss Joan Mulligan, and Robert Benoliel.

To Fred Davis, Virginia Olesen, and Elvi Whittaker I express appreciation for the data provided by the Nursing Careers Project (USPHS Grant NU00024). I wish also to thank the publishers of *The American Scholar* and Wayne Dodd for permission to reprint his poem "Not the Dying," originally appearing in *The American Scholar*, 34 (Summer, 1965), p. 430.

To the students and faculties who provided the data, I am especially grateful for their willingness to make themselves and their institutions available to me. For their cooperation and courage, I am indebted to the following schools: St. Francis Memorial Hospital School of Nursing, San Francisco; St. Joseph College of Nursing, San Francisco; St. Luke's Hospital School of Nursing, San Francisco; Highland School of Nursing, Oakland; and the School of Nursing, University of California Medical Center, San Francisco.

In appreciation for their clerical and editorial assistance, and for their patience, I wish especially to thank Mrs. Bess Sonoda Chang, Mrs. Kathleen Williams, and Mrs. Elaine McLarin.

J. C. Q.

Contents

The Nurse and the Dying Patient

| Chapter 1 | The Student, the School, and the Problem of Death |

Death is one of the basic features of human existence, yet in twentieth-century American society young people are exposed to a strange paradox. On the one hand, they see violent death presented in brutal detail on television and in films. On the other, they have little opportunity to participate directly in the mourning process and family rituals which were relatively common in the home some fifty years ago.[1] According to some social scientists, death has become a taboo topic, and many activities formerly performed by the family at the time of death have now been assumed by special functionaries. Furthermore, those who are dying or are reminders of death, like the aged, tend to be segregated from the rest of society.[2] Dying has become more and more isolated from everyday life.[3]

[1] The close family involvement in these matters has been described by James Agee in *A Death in the Family* (New York: Avon, 1957).

[2] Herman Feifel, "Death," *Taboo Topics*, in Norman L. Farberow, ed. (New York: Atherton, 1963), pp. 8–21; Robert Fulton, *"Death and the Self,"* *Journal of Religion and Health*, 3 (July, 1964), pp. 359–368.

[3] In a similar way, the process of birth has moved from the home into

As changes in medical technology have altered the characters of hospitals and the patient populations who reside therein, so also have public health measures and improvements in preventive medicine produced a decrease in death from infection—particularly among younger persons in the society. In the middle-class urban home of today, death has become an uncommon incident. By comparison, in the nineteenth century it was a rare individual who had not seen dying at home and had not participated directly in the funeral and mourning activities which followed.[4] Close personal encounters with dying are no longer commonplace during the growing-up process. Unlike those who entered medicine and nursing at the turn of the century, young people entering these fields today have had little personal experience with death. Yet they have chosen occupations which carry a direct responsibility for protecting the populace from death for as long as is possible.

This book reports on the impact and meaning of death in the ongoing life of the young woman who is becoming a nurse.[5] More specifically, the book describes some attitudes and actions of these professionals-in-training when they are brought into contact with dying, a significant human experience which has become hidden or disguised by the society in which they live. The book does not solely describe "attitudes toward death," however. It is more directly concerned with the process whereby nurse students learn particular ways of dealing with dying patients. Reflecting a sociological perspective, the book portrays the school of nursing as a socializing agency which introduces the students to a set of customs, beliefs, and practices about death.

the hospital, with the result that young people no longer see the beginning and the ending of life incorporated into their everyday patterns of living. For the nurse student, being present during the birth of a child can be as significant a personal experience as being present at the time of a death.

[4] Geoffrey Gorer, "The Pornography of Death," *Identity and Anxiety*, in Maurice R. Stein, Arthur J. Vidich, and David Manning White, eds. (New York: Free Press, 1960), pp. 402–407.

[5] Although there are increasing numbers of men entering the field of nursing, the study focused only on women students.

This book came into being as part of a larger study of how nursing and medical personnel give care to dying patients.[6] In a recently published volume, Glaser and Strauss have identified some recurrent patterns of interaction which take place between dying patients and those who work in hospitals, and have described some serious decisions and emotionally distressing problems which nurses confront when they work around these patients.[7] Glaser and Strauss have observed further that hospital personnel who are in contact with terminal patients are often disturbed by their own ineptness in handling the dying patient and his family. The evidence they present seems clear—provision of care for the dying is not an easy task for many nurses. Direct questioning of nurses with varied educational and experiential backgrounds supported this premise and also suggested that the educational preparation offered by many schools of nursing does not adequately prepare beginning nurses for the work realities and serious decisions that they soon face in the hospital.

Interviews with newly graduated nurses from many different parts of the United States indicated that the preparation offered to nurse students with respect to care for the dying was far from standardized. Some nurses reported little or no experience with death during their days as students. Others described many experiences with dying patients—sometimes under very positive circumstances, but often not. The variation in reported experience suggested that what students learn about the care of dying patients takes place as much by chance as by advance planning and that schools of nursing give relatively little consistent attention to teaching about death, and particularly to the interactional problems associated with the dying process.

[6] The investigation began in 1961 and was supported by Public Health Service Research Grant No. NU–00047 from the Division of Nursing, Bureau of State Services-Community Health. Directed by Anselm L. Strauss, the project was conducted at the School of Nursing, University of California Medical Center, San Francisco, California. The members of the research team were Jeanne C. Quint and Barney G. Glaser.

[7] Barney G. Glaser and Anselm L. Strauss, *Awareness of Dying* (Chicago: Aldine, 1965).

The questions began to take form. *How does the education of nurse students prepare them to cope with what is obviously a difficult nursing problem? What are they taught about death, and when? Under what circumstances are they assigned to dying patients? What are the consequences for students when the assignment takes place during the first year in school?—at a later time? What do the students consider important in the care of dying patients? What situations give them pleasure? What situations cause them difficulty? How is the care of the dying patient incorporated into the developing nurse identity? How does the social structure of the nursing school determine when and how the students are likely to encounter dying patients?* In seeking answers to these questions the investigator turned directly to schools of nursing.

The material for this book is derived from data collected in five schools of nursing in the Bay Area of San Francisco. Schools with organizational differences were chosen for comparative purposes—to enable the investigator to observe what happened to the students under different teaching conditions and in a variety of hospital locales. One school was administered by a university and offered both graduate and undergraduate programs in nursing. The other four were administered by hospitals and were chosen for their diversity in organizational structure and in type of hospital. The data were obtained primarily through unstructured interviews with students and teachers, although field work (a combination of observation and interviewing) was used to some extent. A detailed description of the methods used for data collection and analysis is given in Appendix A. Reflecting the exploratory nature of the study, the research design was a loose one, deliberately chosen to provide a flexible approach to a difficult problem.

The theoretical orientation came from three converging themes —the development of identity, the school as a socializing agency, and bereavement behavior as a culturally derived phenomenon. The students and the schools were viewed as products of a society with a particular orientation toward death. Both had the values, beliefs, and practices of Western culture concerning human death.

Development of Identity, Educational Socialization, Bereavement

The research problem was viewed within the framework of symbolic interaction theory which assumes that human behavior and appraisal of the self are shaped and controlled (and altered) through interactions with other persons.[8] The assumption was made that encounters with dying persons were likely to be significant incidents if only because of the negative values associated with death in the Western culture. The assumption was not made that these incidents would *necessarily* be negative experiences for the students. Rather it was important to keep an open view on the meaning these experiences had for students. From the many concepts and ideas formulated within the symbolic interaction framework, the concept of turning points was selected for use in this analysis. Turning points are viewed as critical incidents which cause a person to recognize that he is not the same as before. They occur as junctures during the process of identity development or transformation.[9] The concept of turning points was particularly useful for considering the impact of various types of encounters with death as they impinged on young women who were in the process of developing a new identity—that of nurse.

The development of the new identity was part of their socialization both to nursing and to the highly complex hospital organization. The socialization process experienced by the students took place within an educational institution.[10] The circumstances un-

---

[8] See Howard S. Becker, et al., *Boys in White* (Chicago: University of Chicago Press, 1961), pp. 17–48; Anselm L. Strauss, *Mirrors and Masks: The Search For Identity* (New York: Free Press, 1959), pp. 44–88; and Arnold Rose, ed., *Human Behavior and Social Processes* (Boston: Houghton Mifflin, 1962).

[9] Strauss, *op. cit.*, pp. 93–100.

[10] *Socialization* refers to a process whereby an individual learns to perform in a given role.

der which the students actually encountered death were influenced by the social structure and ideology of both the school and the hospital.[11] Stated differently, the student perspective on death was influenced by the culture of the school and the culture of the hospital.[12] As will become clear in subsequent chapters, the meaning of incidents involving death, from the viewpoint of the nurse student, requires some understanding of the context in which the incidents take place.

Finally, both the individuals themselves and the institutions in which they interacted are part of a society in which the socioemotional vulnerability of individuals in bereavement (loss through death) is extremely high. This high vulnerability is directly related to the American small-family system, which leads to a self-involvement with and an emotional attachment to a few select persons, thereby maximizing their psychological significance and making their loss through death almost irreplaceable, psychologically speaking.[13] The American cultural emphasis on loss in bereavement fosters a social role (bereaved person) preoccupied with grief expression but often without socially sanctioned outlets for other strong emotions. The students, their teachers, the hospital staff, and the patients had all absorbed a cultural orientation in which grief and bereavement carry some common expectations and meanings. Grief (feelings of mental suffering or sorrow) is an individual, internalized response, and thus is difficult to ob-

[11] *Ideology* refers to the body of doctrine, myth, and symbols which underlies the operation of an institution or social movement.

[12] Becker, *op. cit.*, p. 34, describes *perspective* "to refer to a co-ordinated set of ideas and actions a person uses in dealing with some problematic situation, to refer to a person's ordinary way of thinking and feeling about and acting in such a situation."

[13] The relationship among social roles with respect to bereavement and cultural values, beliefs, and practices has been conceptualized by Edmund H. Volkart and Stanley T. Michael in "Bereavement and Mental Health," *Explorations in Social Psychiatry* (New York: Basic Books, 1957), pp. 281–307. According to this conceptualization, the development of bereavement behaviors is related to the development of self within a given kind of family structure. The psychological vulnerability of Americans in bereavement is generally high because the culture offers no easy solution to the problem of replacement.

serve. By comparison, bereavement behavior—in the form of a socially sanctioned role with specific social obligations—can be observed and recorded.[14] Under some conditions a student experienced grief and feelings of loss when a patient died. At this point she found herself in a received role—that of bereaved person— but usually without social sanctions for playing the role. A tension existed between the social role of bereaved person and the emergent role of nurse. The relative importance of culturally endowed attitudes and behaviors in response to the loss of a significant person through death served as a frame of reference against which to compare the students' reactions and actions with respect to the deaths of certain of their patients.

Student Experience and the School of Nursing

This book focuses primarily on what happens to the nurse student when she encounters dying patients in the course of learning to be a nurse. In an indirect sense the book is concerned with what happens to dying patients in hospitals, because nurses hold key positions for determining how these patients will live through their final days. The evidence to be presented in forthcoming chapters supports the premise that newly graduated nurses are not well prepared for the work they will be expected to do when they provide care for those who are dying. This result does not reflect the intent of schools of nursing but rather suggests that the magnitude and nature of the problem has not been sufficiently recognized by those responsible for teaching nurses, or, for that matter, by the public at large. The provision of care for those who are dying is a delicate and serious matter. To judge from the data on which this book is based, giving this care is tension-producing for teacher and student alike.

[14] In this society, with its heavy emphasis on loss and the general expectation of grief, a distinction between the concepts of "grief" and "bereavement" has not always been made by psychiatrists and social scientists in describing human behaviors in response to death. In a sense, these writers reflect the cultural assumption that the bereaved person "ought to" show grief. *Ibid.*, pp. 289–290.

The context in which nurse students are assigned to dying patients is described in the next two chapters. The discussion in Chapter 2 centers on the school's instructional program as a whole, with particular attention given to those assignment characteristics which significantly influence when and how students are likely to encounter dying patients. Chapter 3 is more directly concerned with the influence of the individual teacher and considers the relevance of different types of teacher perspectives on death and on teaching. Also described are some of the problems that the dying patient poses for teachers, as well as some work conditions which contribute additional problems for those who teach on the hospital wards.

Chapters 4 and 5 describe the two situations which contribute to significant and meaningful experiences for the students. The relative importance of conversations with dying patients, as well as the various circumstances under which these events take place, is considered in Chapter 4. Sometimes these conversations pose no problems at all. At other times the circumstances can be such that the conversations are extremely difficult and tension-producing. The relationship between the students' awareness of dying and both nondifficult and difficult conversations is considered in detail. Chapter 5 is concerned with the impact of student encounters with death itself, the conditions under which the experiences take place, and the "positive" and "negative" outcomes of these experiences. The impact and meaning of the events is considered from three perspectives—the individual (the human person), the nurse, and the student. Special attention is given to those events that the students describe as troublesome. The chapter ends with a discussion of the aftermath of serious and meaningful encounters with death. Both chapters are primarily concerned with students' reactions and responses to significant experiences involving dying patients. Both chapters also include some immediate and long-term results of these significant experiences.

The discussion in Chapter 6 focuses on the meaning of these events in a different way. The chapter begins by considering how the nurse student acquires some expectations about dying and then incorporates these expectations into a nurse identity primarily committed to recovery care. The chapter then describes what the beginning staff nurse in the hospital learns about dying that may be different from what she learned as a student. Finally, the discussion turns to the conflicts in identity experienced by graduate nurse students when they are put into new kinds of role relationships with dying patients. Essentially, this chapter is concerned with the issue of how to achieve gratification from a work situation (the dying patient) which provides few opportunities to obtain rewards and satisfaction because the demands of the situation are often in conflict with the primary purpose for being a nurse—namely, helping people get well.

Turning away from the nurse's perspective on dying, Chapter 7 deals with what happens to patients and, to a lesser extent, their families when they are brought into contact with nurse students. Frequently the students provide meaningful experiences for dying patients without themselves being aware that they have done so. However, the students can also knowingly influence what happens to these patients. The chapter describes both the positive and the less positive results of assigning dying patients to the students.

The book closes with a chapter addressed to the need for change in schools of nursing if nurses are to be better prepared to provide care for patients who are dying. Provision of this care in hospitals is a very serious and difficult problem, and nurses play a central part in determining what that care will be. The proposals for change became clear only after thoughtful consideration of the findings discussed in previous chapters. They are presented in full recognition that the initiation of changes in nursing practice is neither an easy task nor one to be taken lightly.

This book is written primarily for nurse teachers, practitioners, and students—in the hope that it will help them to take a fresh look at a difficult nursing problem. It may also have value for those who are interested in the sociology of work and in the education of professionals, particularly for those aspects of work which might be called the problem areas or "dirty work." [15] In a very real sense the book is written for all who are concerned with the problem of providing persons who are dying with opportunities to move through their final moments in dignity and with a sense of participation in their deaths.

When reading the book it is well to remember that the persons involved—students, teachers, and patients—are members of a society in which dying is a taboo topic. Furthermore, the same taboos have influenced the development of the social institutions in which nurses practice and are taught. Although nursing is an occupation which has not been isolated from death, as is true of many other fields of work, nonetheless nursing reflects the values, beliefs, and practices of the wider society in which it is immersed.[16]

Nurses and the Problem of Death

Nurses have always had to deal with death because sick patients do not always recover. Thus schools of nursing have had to provide some kind of training for the task. That many staff nurses in hospitals feel ill prepared to cope with the problems of dying patients, and derive little personal satisfaction from these assignments, suggests that schools of nursing have provided insufficient training—particularly in the "hows" of performing the delicate psychological tasks associated with the dying process.[17] To judge from the content of standard nursing textbooks, which contain relatively little about the care of those who are dying,

[15] Everett C. Hughes in *Men and Their Work* (New York: Free Press, 1958), pp. 68–77, talks about the division of labor within professions, such that some have "prestige work" whereas others perform "dirty work."

[16] Fulton, *op. cit.*, p. 360, presents the viewpoint that in contemporary America, death is treated like a communicable disease—something to be *hidden* from daily living.

[17] Robert Fulton and Phyllis A. Langton in "Attitudes Toward Death: An Emerging Mental Health Problem," *Nursing Forum*, Vol. 3, No. 1 (1964), pp. 105–112, have considered how the culture's conflicting concepts about death have contributed to the problems which nurses face in dealing with dying patients and their families.

nurses have been mainly concerned with the life-saving aspects of nursing practice. The Harmer and Henderson classic, for example, devoted ten pages out of a total of 1,008 to the care of the dying.[18] Moreover, the content quite specifically centered on the practices to be used by nurses when the patient is near the point of death and on the procedures to follow in disposing of the body. It seems likely that nursing textbooks mirror the emphasis given by schools of nursing to teaching the care of the dying, both with respect to the content deemed to be important and the amount of time allotted to the topic.[19]

A perusal of nursing periodicals reveals little evidence that care of the dying was ever a major concern of nurses in this country. The *Cumulative Indexes* of the *American Journal of Nursing* between 1900 and 1960 list twenty-one articles dealing with death and dying, another eighteen concerning mortality rates.[20] In comparison with the total number of articles printed during the sixty years, those dealing with death were few indeed and focused mainly on the nursing practices to be employed during the final stages of life. Like the wider society of which it was a part, the nursing world gave scant attention to the social and psychological aspects of death, and instead focused mainly on the technical matters which nurses were expected to perform when their patients died. Only recently have the nursing journals demonstrated a shift in emphasis, evidenced by an increase in articles devoted to the psychological aspects of care of the dying.[21] This greater concern with death is not unique to nursing, however, and a sim-

[18] Bertha Harmer and Virginia Henderson, *Textbook of the Principles and Practice of Nursing,* 4th ed. (New York: Macmillan, 1939), pp. 411–420.

[19] Other nursing textbooks showed a similar amount of space devoted to care of the dying, in proportion to the other topics covered. Among those examined were Mildred L. Montag and Margaret Filson, *Nursing Arts,* 2nd ed. (Philadelphia: Saunders, 1953); Alice L. Price, *The Art, Science and Spirit of Nursing,* 2nd ed. (Philadelphia: Saunders, 1954); Lulu W. Wolf, *Nursing* (New York: Appleton-Century-Crofts, 1947).

[20] *Cumulative Indexes, American Journal of Nursing,* Vol. 1–60 (October, 1900–December, 1960).

[21] This trend began with "The Nurse and the Dying Patient," by Catherine M. Norris in *American Journal of Nursing,* 55 (October, 1955), pp. 1214–1217.

ilar increase in books and articles about death and dying can be found in the social and medical science literature in general.[22] The popular literature has not been exempt from the movement and has included publications of a philosophical nature and others with pragmatic and enlightening aims.[23] Many publications reflect an increasing concern with the moral, legal, religious, and personal issues associated with a changing picture of death in this country.[24]

Social change and scientific advance in the twentieth century have made the problems related to death increasingly complex for those who enter the healing professions. People are living longer. With an aging population has come an increase in the chronic diseases, such as cancer and heart disease. Because improvements in symptomatic medical therapy prolong the condition of living with diseases which formerly were rapidly fatal, persons with such diseases are often in and out of the hospital several times before death occurs.

Medical technology has radically changed the character of dying as a hospital problem in other ways as well. Persons with diseases carrying a fatal connotation are now hospitalized for diagnostic and treatment procedures which require complex equip-

[22] See Herman Feifel, ed., *The Meaning of Death* (New York: Blakiston, 1959); Margaretta K. Bowers, et al., *Counseling the Dying* (New York: Thomas Nelson, 1964); Robert Fulton, ed., *Death and Identity* (New York: Wiley, 1965).

[23] Cyrus Sulzberger, *My Brother Death* (New York: Harper, 1961); Jacques Choron, *Death and Western Thought* (New York: Collier Books, 1963); and Jessica Mitford, *The American Way of Death* (New York: Simon and Schuster, 1963) are among the recent publications.

[24] Frank J. Ayd, Jr., "The Hopeless Case," *Journal of the American Medical Association*, 181 (September 29, 1962), pp. 1099–1102; Otto E. Guttentag, "The Meaning of Death in Medical Theory," *Stanford Medical Bulletin*, 17 (August, 1959), pp. 165–170; Louis Lasagna, *The Doctors' Dilemmas* (New York: Harper, 1962); Adriaan Verwoerdt, "Communication with the Fatally Ill," *CA, A Cancer Journal for Clinicians* (May–June, 1965), pp. 105–111 are representative of the trend. Some publications are addressed specifically to the clergy, for example, Carl J. Scherzer, *Ministering to the Dying* (Englewood Cliffs, N.J.: Prentice-Hall, 1963), and C. E. Benda, "Bereavement and Grief Work," *Journal of Pastoral Care*, 16 (1962), pp. 1–13.

ment and the specialized skills of trained technicians. Changes in surgical and anesthetic techniques have greatly increased the numbers of hazardous operations performed—particularly in large urban hospitals and research centers. Patients enter these hospitals for such complicated treatments as kidney transplants or extensive cardiac surgery, where the risks are high and the chances for recovery are somewhat unpredictable. Not all patients who consent to these treatments can be expected to survive. In some hospital wards nurses today are providing care for large numbers of patients who are dying or who face the possibility of imminent death.

Scientific and engineering discoveries have had a profound effect on treatment of the dying through the development of techniques and machines which can be used to extend life. The question of deciding when a person is dead has become more complicated since the advent of many new life-preserving measures. There has also been a marked increase in the use of heroic measures, particularly by younger physicians.[25] Life-prolonging equipment gives the physician greater control over postponing the patient's death but can also make for complex and difficult decisions.[26] The issue of prolonging life when recovery is no longer possible is a serious one, and has led to statements by religious authorities and concerned laymen.[27] Both the Roman Catholic Church and the Jewish law oppose euthanasia (active steps to hasten death), but both sanction the withdrawal of any factor which may artificially

[25] Heroic measures are the speedy and all-out efforts made to stave off death when one of the body's vital systems suddenly fails, e.g., the heart stops beating and external cardiac massage is applied. Titled "Code 99!" a description of "hospital heroics" in action was made in *Life*, 56 (February 28, 1964), pp. 52b–61.

[26] See Glaser and Strauss, *op. cit.*, pp. 194–203, for a discussion of the medical problem of prolonging life. See also James A. Knight, "Philosophic Implications of Terminal Illness," *North Carolina Medical Journal*, 22 (1961), pp. 493–495; Lawrence A. Kohn, "Thoughts on the Care of the Hopelessly Ill," *Medical Times*, 89 (1961), pp. 1177–1181; T. T. Jones, "Dignity in Death: The Application and Withholding of Interventive Measures," *Journal of the Louisiana Medical Society* (1961), pp. 180–183.

[27] Joseph Fletcher, "The Patient's Right to Die," *Harper's*, 221 (October, 1960), pp. 139–143.

delay death when the person is known to be dying.[28] That physicians must make this type of decision is well recognized. It is less popularly known that nurses who take care of dying patients are often in situations where decisions relative to these matters are made. Although nurses may not emphasize this facet of their practice, the fact remains that those who work in hospitals must meet and decide about many delicate problems associated with the dying process.

Within three medical specialties—psychiatry, geriatrics, and pediatrics—there are indications of increasing concern with the problems of grief and bereavement.[29] Recent nursing publications which have focused on the care of the dying reflect the psychiatric influence, with an emphasis on the nurse's responsibility for providing emotional support for the individual and for his family.[30] Nurse writers have addressed far less attention to the work realities and specific decisions that are imposed on nurses because of the way that work in the hospital is organized.[31] The personalized

[28] See Pope Pius XII, allocution delivered to the International Congress of Anesthesiologists, November 24, 1957 and published in *Acta Apostolica Sedis*, 49 (1957), pp. 1027–1033; Rabbi Immanuel Jakobovits, "The Dying and Their Treatment in Jewish Law: Preparation for Death and Euthanasia," *The Hebrew Medical Journal* (*Harofé Haivri*), 2 (1961), pp. 251–242.

[29] See "Part 3. Grief and Mourning: The Reaction to Death," in Robert Fulton, ed., *Death and Identity* (New York: Wiley, 1965), pp. 181–329. In the *Journal of Human Relations*, 13 (1965), pp. 118–141, Richard A. Kalish has listed a 370-item bibliography on death and bereavement.

[30] Some examples are Jeanne E. Blumberg and Eleanor E. Drummond, *Nursing Care of the Long-Term Patient* (New York: Springer, 1963), pp. 95–112; Gertrud Bertrand Ujhely, *The Nurse and Her Problem Patients* (New York: Springer, 1963), pp. 41–48; George L. Engel, "Grief and Grieving," *American Journal of Nursing*, 64 (September, 1964), pp. 93–98; Richard A. Kalish, "Dealing with the Grieving Family," *RN*, 26 (May, 1963), pp. 81–84; Sister M. Willa Kyle, "The Nurse's Approach to the Patient Attempting to Adjust to Inoperable Cancer," *Convention Clinical Sessions, Vol. 8: Effective Therapeutic Communication in Nursing* (New York: American Nurses' Association, 1964), pp. 27–39; Sylvia J. Bruce, "Reactions of Nurses and Mothers to Stillbirths," *Nursing Outlook*, 10 (February, 1962), pp. 88–91.

[31] The complexity of the large general hospital is described by Robert N. Wilson in "The Social Structure of a General Hospital," *The Annals of the American Academy of Political and Social Science*, 346 (March, 1963), pp. 67–76.

and comforting care created by Dr. Cicely Saunders in a small London hospital for patients dying of cancer is difficult to achieve in the busy recovery-focused atmosphere of a large, modern hospital.[32] Within the latter settings it is the nursing staff which carries major responsibility for providing comfort care when the recovery goal is no longer possible.[33]

Within the last twenty-five years the provision of care for the dying has become an increasingly complex hospital phenomenon, and nurses are faced with many situations which are both problematic and distressing. At the same time, those who are entering the field have had few opportunities to face death as a significant part of their personal life experience. In this alone they come less well prepared than their predecessors at the turn of the century. In addition to these changes—both closely related to the changing picture of death in American life—the society is changing in other ways as well. As is also true with the other health professions, nursing is being modified by many social forces which are producing changes in the kind and quantity of nursing services.

The public demand for better health care and services increased rapidly following the Second World War. In 1948 the six national nursing organizations joined forces to consider what might be done to meet these new demands.[34] Pressures for the expansion and improvement of nursing services, in turn, led to changes in the education of those engaging in providing these services. The impetus for educational reform came from within the nursing profession itself and contributed to organizational and instructional changes in many schools of nursing.

Social Change and the Education of Nurses

Through its national nursing organizations, the nursing profession in 1948 set up a joint committee to develop programs for the improvement of nursing services. The committee's first task

[32] Cicely Saunders, "The Last Stages of Life," *American Journal of Nursing*, 65 (March, 1965), pp. 70–75.

[33] Glaser and Strauss, *op. cit.*, pp. 204–225.

[34] *Nursing Schools at the Mid-Century* (New York: National Committee for the Improvement of Nursing Services, 1950), p. xiii.

was to examine current practices in basic nursing education, and an evaluation of these practices was published in 1950.[35] An interim classification of nursing schools included in that report served as a stimulus for the elimination of apprentice-type training. Organized nursing began an active campaign to improve nursing curricula.[36] Pressures for change were exerted upon hospital schools, the principal source from which professional nurses are drawn, but questions were also posed about the curricula of nursing schools affiliated with universities and colleges. Preparation for degree programs was found to be highly variable and, in some instances, inferior to that offered in some hospital schools.[37] The reform movement exerted pressure for self-improvement on all schools of nursing through the establishment of a national accreditation program sponsored by the National League for Nursing.

A second outcome of the educational reform movement was an increase in curriculum experimentation. The concern with curriculum experimentation caused changes in already established nursing programs, but also contributed to the development of new and sometimes controversial educational ventures.[38] Increased importance was assigned to clinical nursing and to the instructor's role in planning learning experiences for nurse students.[39] Experimentation with clinical teaching methods began in the university schools, but the influence of new and varied teaching techniques also reached into other schools of nursing by means of publication in nursing periodicals and by the persuasiveness of

[35] *Ibid.*

[36] In commenting on the conditions in nursing education, Esther Lucille Brown in *Nursing for the Future* (New York: Russell Sage Foundation, 1948), p. 48, had noted, "In spite of improvements that have been made in most schools over the years, it remains apprentice training."

[37] Margaret Bridgman, *Collegiate Education for Nursing* (New York: Russell Sage Foundation, 1953), p. 96.

[38] Mildred L. Montag, *The Education of Nursing Technicians* (New York: Putnam's, 1951). See also the section "Baccalaureate Programs for Nursing Education" in *The Yearbook of Modern Nursing 1957–58* (New York: Putnam's, 1958), pp. 275–297.

[39] Sister M. Thomas Kolba, "Teaching Clinical Nursing," *The Yearbook of Modern Nursing 1956* (New York: Putnam's, 1956), pp. 255–259.

nurse teachers who had been trained to use the newer approaches.

During the postwar period, nursing education was greatly influenced by the growing mental health movement. Increased importance was attached by many nurse educators to the psychological aspects of nursing care. The nurse was perceived as a dynamic agent of change in her interactions with patients, and "fostering personality development in the direction of maturity" was viewed as a function of nursing and of nursing education.[40] The psychiatric perspective became a persuasive force in determining both the content of nursing courses and the teaching practices to be utilized, particularly with respect to clinical practice. Again, the psychological emphasis made its greatest impact in collegiate programs, but teaching about communication skills and the nurse-patient relationship spread into nursing curricula at all levels of education. Recent articles concerned with teaching students about the care of dying patients also reflect the psychiatric perspective.[41]

Curriculum experimentation, accreditation pressures, and a growing emphasis on psychological nursing care were significant forces for change in schools of nursing during the 1950's. In California, for example, psychiatric clinical experience became a state requirement for graduation from professional nursing schools in 1957.[42] Stimulated by the pioneer ventures of experimental educational programs, some nurse educators made a sharp break with the past. One modification involved a shift from using the traditional hospital work assignment to a selective use of hospital pa-

[40] Hildegard E. Peplau, *Interpersonal Relations in Nursing* (New York: Putnam's, 1952), p. xii.

[41] Marilyn Folck and Phyllis Nie, "Nursing Students Learn to Face Death," *Nursing Outlook*, 7 (1959), pp. 510–513; Eleanor Drummond and Jeanne Blumberg, "Death and the Curriculum," *Journal of Nursing Education*, 1 (May–June, 1962), pp. 21–28; Berniece M. Wagner, "Teaching Students to Work with the Dying," *American Journal of Nursing*, 64 (November, 1964), pp. 128–131.

[42] Specifically, "an applicant who entered on or before August 1, 1952 but who graduated (completed) on or before September 10, 1957 must show satisfactory evidence of . . . 12 weeks psychiatric clinical experience." Statement on Credentials, Board of Nursing Education and Nurse Registration, State of California, revised January 20, 1965, p. 3.

tients during short and well-supervised practice periods. The ideology of professional nursing practice was undergoing a change in emphasis which, in turn, was effecting changes in the teaching of nurses. Within many schools of nursing, new assignment patterns were evolving under the influence of changing social conditions. This point is an important one because what students learn about death and the care of dying patients, as well as how they learn it, is greatly affected by the conditions under which patients are used as school assignments.

It should now be abundantly clear that this book is concerned with a cultural phenomenon. In reading the chapters which follow, it is well to remember that the persons involved and the institutions in which they are functioning are part of a society in which the subject of dying has been something of a forbidden topic. Conversation about dying and death can cause personal discomfort for individuals not accustomed to such discussion. So too can reading about these subjects when they are personally meaningful. For those who have had little direct experience with death and hospital life, the incidents described in the book may sometimes come as a surprise. For nurses they are likely to trigger memories of personal encounters with death, particularly those which occurred while they were students. The reader is warned that what is reported here will not always provide easy or comfortable reading. The chapter which follows considers how the general silence about dying has influenced instructional programs in schools of nursing, thereby profoundly affecting what happens to nurse students when they are assigned to dying patients. The chapter provides a contextual framework for understanding the critical incidents and meaningful experiences which are described later.

Chapter 2 | Dying Patients, Death, and the Curriculum

When and how nurse students encounter dying patients and what they are taught about death depends on several factors—the ideology of the school, the organization of course work and practice opportunities, the rationale underlying the use of patients as assignments, the settings used for practice, and the approaches used to teach about the care of dying patients. More particularly, this chapter is concerned with two effects of the instructional program: how it contributes to the student perspective on *what is important* in providing care for dying patients, and how it determines the kinds of encounters students are likely to have with dying patients.

The analysis on which the chapter is based began as a comparison of the undergraduate instructional program in the university school and the programs offered by the schools affiliated with hospitals. The teaching programs of the five schools were observed to be similar in many ways, but variable in others. It soon became evident that the curricula were very similar with respect to the subject matter related to death, the organization of course work and practice opportunities, and some standardized teaching practices (including supervisory techniques) commonly used in the hospital locale. These curriculum similarities and their effects on the students are considered first.

The Curriculum Emphasis on Life-Saving Goals

In all of the schools the curricula stressed the life-saving goals of nursing practice. Nursing courses gave priority to the nurse's responsibilities for helping patients recover from illness or adjust to changes in daily living. The changes requiring adjustment in daily living were of many sorts, from a new baby in the family to a chronic incapacitating physical or mental disability. Relatively little attention was directed toward the nurse's responsibilities or problems in caring for those patients who face death rather than recovery.

A limited concern with dying was revealed in several ways. Class discussions on nursing responsibility with respect to care for the dying were usually scheduled near the end of a course. Not uncommonly, a beginning instructor was given the responsibility for conducting the discussion. The content presented was generally limited to four fundamental activities: observing for changes in physical signs and symptoms and reporting these to the physician; providing comfort and relief from pain for the dying patient; calling a minister or priest when the possibility of death became apparent; and providing support and comfort for the family through the dying period (in pediatric nursing the management of grief-stricken families was emphasized). In general, the content focused on the nurse's role in providing care for a person near the point of death. The teachers emphasized those matters for which the nurse could be held accountable—by law, by hospital regulation, or by moral and ethical interpretations of personal responsibility.[1]

---

[1] In a heterogeneous society the moral and ethical basis for action is not always clear-cut in matters concerned with death. The sources for individual

In some of the schools, but not all, a panel of clergymen representing three major religions—Roman Catholic, Protestant, and Judaic—discussed religious practices as they pertained to those who were dying.

Not only was the subject matter related to death somewhat limited in scope, but none of the schools had an organized and coordinated plan for ensuring that every student was assigned to a dying patient (through the period of death) while in school. Those students who had a carefully planned assignment to a dying patient had it because of the interest and concern of a particular teacher. A concerned teacher tried to arrange assignments to dying patients for all students while they were under her direction, but she often could not guarantee the experience because of the limited time available.

Although many nurse teachers expressed the opinion that students probably "should have" experience with dying patients, their individual and collective behaviors supported the primacy of recovery goals. Within their individual work spheres most teachers stressed the importance of helping patients get well, and patient assignments were made with this orientation in mind. The teachers selected the patients because they had certain diagnoses or because they provided the opportunity for practice in performing procedures. Procedures might be technical, interpersonal, or a combination of both.

It would be inaccurate to say that no attention was given to teaching about nursing actions in the face of death. What the teachers emphasized came from a perspective that dying is a situation which demands responsible professional performance by the nurse. That is, there are prescribed behaviors which the nurse is expected to use when a patient dies or is facing imminent death. The nurse perspective on dying is one concerned with safe and adequate performance.

---

decision making lie in the tenets of religion, the society, the family, and the medical and nursing professions. In discussing these matters with the students, the teachers must necessarily interpret "right behavior" in terms of their own personal perspectives on the issue.

The Nurse Perspective on Care of the Dying

From the viewpoint of the nurse, there are two kinds of death encounters which are significant. First, there are those in which death is medically accepted and is recognized as inevitable. Death is expected although the estimates of the time of its occurrence may be more or less certain, depending on the individual's understanding of what is happening.[2] Second, there are encounters where the possibility of imminent death appears suddenly. In such cases heroic means are brought into play in an effort to prevent the unexpected death from taking place. Emergencies can occur anywhere in the hospital but are *anticipated* in some settings because the medical conditions under treatment there precipitate emergencies with great frequency.

The standards and expectations governing acceptable nurse performance when death is expected are different from those required when the unexpected prospect of death arises. (There can be an overlapping of functioning in specific situations, as when the patient known to be dying develops a complication which requires emergency treatment.) The nurse is confronted with somewhat different sets of problems, and timing and judgment are the critical variants which influence decisions to be made and actions to be taken.

When death appears inevitable, the nurse is responsible for minimizing the patient's physical discomfort, providing him relief from pain and implementing those medical tasks which the physician has delegated to her. Her principal goal is the provision of care and comfort until the patient dies, and she often must provide support for the grieving family. The nurse in this situation is expected to perform a variety of activities: providing personal care which the sick person cannot perform for himself (this requires a direct handling of the person's body); conversing with the patient, as determined by his state of consciousness and by

[2] For a discussion of what is involved in defining a person as dying see Barney G. Glaser and Anselm L. Strauss, *Awareness of Dying* (Chicago: Aldine, 1965), pp. 16–26.

his wishes; using medical equipment as required, with skill and sureness; watching for changes in the patient's condition; recognizing when pain medication or sedation is needed; effecting such treatments as have been ordered by the physician; and calling the doctor at an appropriate time. (Sometimes the doctor is called when death is approaching, and sometimes when he is needed to pronounce the patient deceased. In practice, the decision as to when to notify the doctor depends on the kind of working relationship which exists between the particular physician and the nursing staff.) In addition, there are various hospital and legal routines that are required for body handling and disposal before the nurse can consider the assignment officially completed.

The emergency is a sharp contrast. The possibility of death appears precipitously, with little warning, and the situation requires rapid judgments concerning what needs to be done. Whether the emergency be hemorrhage or cardiac arrest, successful performance depends on the following activities: recognizing the situation and its urgency; initiating a call for the physician's help; performing appropriate emergency actions until the doctor arrives; collecting and organizing equipment as required; and assisting the physician(s) until the crisis has been averted. Time is a crucial factor in an emergency, and speed in decision making may make the difference between a life saved and a life lost. Time is of little importance, however, without proper diagnosis of the situation and the initiation of appropriate and helpful assistance. The heroic situation has two possible outcomes, usually accompanied by somewhat different reactions. In general, when a life has been saved, the nurse reaction is one of accomplishment. When a life has been lost, there are several possible responses—"we did our best"; "we could have done better"; "we made an error in judgment."

The care-and-comfort and the heroic assignments require different performances from the nurse, yet in both instances she carries considerable responsibility for what is happening to another person's life. Teachers of nursing, as well as nurses in general, place a high value on responsible behavior by the nurse.

Some well-defined ways of behaving have come to be generally accepted as standards to be used for judging the actions of nurses in the face of death, and teachers continue to emphasize the importance of these actions.[3] Thus they become standards which carry critical significance for the students who use them to appraise their own behaviors as nurses.

The nurse perspective on death is influential in determining the subject matter which has priority. Some standardized teaching practices determine how much attention is given to teaching about death in the clinical setting. The probabilities that students will actually encounter death is directly related to the planning and patterning of assignments to patients.

Assignment Characteristics and Standardized Teaching Practices

Each of the five schools operated with a prescribed curriculum derived from the school's objectives. Within this framework the students were assigned to a series of clinical practice fields—sometimes within the context of the course itself and sometimes simply concurrent with classwork. The students practiced nursing in many different locales, and they moved about within the hospital and to other settings as well. Whether for a full semester or for a few weeks on a given ward, the nurse student's position was one of constant adjustment to the expectations of different faculty and to the work requirements of different assignment settings.[4] Each instructor had autonomy in making patient assignments and there was little evidence of organized and consistent transmittal of information from teacher to teacher about assignments to patients who represented key nursing problems. In general, a teacher

---

[3] Standards for behavior are generally presented in nursing textbooks as activities which the nurse is expected to perform. For example, there are specific actions deemed necessary in nursing the unconscious patient. See Kathleen Newton Shafer, et al., *Medical-Surgical Nursing* (St. Louis: Mosby, 1958), pp. 100–108.

[4] See Jeanne C. Quint and Anselm L. Strauss, "Nursing Students, Assignments, and Dying Patients," *Nursing Outlook*, 12 (January, 1964), pp. 24–27.

had to rely on the students for information about assignments they had not yet had. Thus the students could, and sometimes did, evade unwanted experiences with dying patients.

For the most part teachers in clinical settings were concerned with many different and time-consuming matters—the safety of assigned patients, the supervision of various numbers of students, cooperation with the hospital staff, and maintenance of records of student performance.[5] Because of their many and varied commitments, the teachers often were unaware of what was happening to the students during the time spent with their patients.

The teachers in clinical settings used several standardized practices whereby the students learned which nursing practices were important. The emphasis given to supervision of student performance in such matters as the giving of medications stressed the danger of making mistakes. A teacher's concerns about preventing these errors is clearly evidenced in the following comment.

Of course, we are always concerned about that. Our students are very closely supervised on medications. They're not allowed to give medications until we are sure they are capable of handling it. They are checked very, very closely on a one-to-one basis. Then the younger students will give medications to their own patients for a long time, and they are spot checked. Then after they are released and told they can go ahead, they are re-spot checked, and frequently to see that they're not getting lax in their procedures. The same with the seniors. When they take over, we like to have them give meds to the whole floor. And they are supervised on a one-to-one basis before we let them do it. We do have medicine mistakes. When we do, we are real concerned about it. The students have to see the director. They have to talk to the instructor. For some reason, I don't know why it is, they realize the importance of it, we've never had any problem with our students not telling as soon as they make a mistake. They are very willing to come out and say, "I did this," instead of trying to hide it or cover up.

[5] A description of the multiple work problems of the clinical teacher is well stated by Agnes P. Mullins in "First Clinical Assignments," *Nursing Outlook*, 13 (February, 1965), pp. 47–50.

The emphasis given to preventing errors in medication strongly affected the students' concerns about their own performances. Making such a mistake tended to result in feelings of "personal failure." A concern about personal negligence (brought from the general culture) was thereby additionally reinforced.[6]

Sometimes one teacher was responsible for course work and another for clinical supervision, with the result that the students had to decide between different expectations about "proper" performance in the care of dying patients. Frequently class demonstrations on such matters as postmortem body care took place long before many students met the problem in the hospital—if they met it at all—while they were students. Many teachers did not initiate discussion about death and dying in ward conferences, but let the students carry the initiative in introducing the topic into these discussions. These generalized teaching practices were influential in two ways. The students placed high value on protecting themselves from negligent performance. They also acquired the feeling that care of the dying was relatively unimportant as a nursing task because their teachers gave little consistent attention to teaching about it.

Rotation of patients was a technique utilized by many teachers in making clinical assignments. Patients who represented meaningful examples of the problems being studied in class were assigned to different students for short periods of time. This teaching technique was designed to provide practice opportunities for as many students as possible when a "good experience" was available. A "good experience" might be a patient with a particular diagnosis or a person having a special treatment. Rotation of patient assignments brought the individual student into limited contact with any one patient. Such brief contacts with patients resulted in the students moving in and out of many relationships with patients without much awareness of the patients' perspectives or future orientations. The students were exposed to bits

[6] The negative connotations associated with individual failure, as a basic theme of the dominant American value system, are discussed by Richard J. Hill in "The Right to Fail," *Nursing Outlook*, 13 (April, 1965), pp. 38–41.

and pieces of the patients' lives, and they learned to focus on segments of nursing care—often without seeing the reality of what was happening to these patients and their families. Because they focused their attention on other matters, students often were unaware that certain of the patients to whom they were assigned were dying.

When and how the student actually encountered dying patients was determined by the context in which patients were used as school assignments. Reflecting a particular philosophy of nursing practice and philosophy of education, the assignment context in each school was characterized by distinct features—the numbers of patients comprising an assignment on a given day, the patient assignment goals, and the amount and kind of supervision offered. Different perspectives on nursing and on the learning process led to different administrative decisions concerning when and how patients were to be used for assignments. Thus a school with a philosophy that nursing care was twenty-four hours of hospital work per day had a different assignment policy than did a school where nursing was viewed principally as a person-to-person relationship which could be offered in many different community settings. The undergraduate and graduate programs in the university school of nursing all reflected the latter viewpoint on nursing. The hospital schools were concerned with preparing nurses to work in hospitals, but the assignment contexts formulated by these schools were not identical—thus students might or might not have assignments involving the death of a patient. In all schools the hospital locale used for practice was an important component of the assignment context.

The Influence of the Hospital Locale

In each school two or more hospitals were used for student experience, but the students had most of their patient assignments in their home hospitals—the hospital with which the school was most closely aligned. The students most commonly encountered death on medical and surgical wards in these home hospitals, but the numbers of deaths in these different institutions varied considerably. The private hospitals had fewer deaths proportionately than did the county hospital or the university medical center, in part because the latter institutions (in addition to being larger) were used for both research and training purposes and contained large numbers of patients with unusual conditions or poor prognoses. In these settings new and dramatic medical therapies were commonplace, and the nurse students were likely to be exposed to situations which were relatively uncommon in private hospitals, such as many high-risk patients and the not infrequent use of heroic life-saving measures.[7]

The extent to which the students actually encountered dying patients and death was influenced by the faculty's selective use of wards within each hospital. Some wards, such as intensive-care units, have high death ratios and a frequent use of heroic treatment, but the time given to assignments on such high-risk wards was often brief. Thus a student might or might not encounter death or an emergency while she was there. (Sometimes hospital policy did not permit students to be assigned in the intensive-care unit.) Similarly, the use of wards with low death frequencies meant that students had limited opportunities for encounters with dying patients simply because the experience was seldom available. By comparison, assignment to a geriatrics ward (or any ward with large numbers of sick, elderly patients) increased the chances of witnessing death and of giving care during the final stages of terminal illness. The school's assignment policy determined which wards were used and therefore determined also the extent to which dying patients were available within the *assignment context*. The probability that students would or would not encounter dying patients, however, was more directly a function of the purpose underlying the use of patients as school assignments.

[7] "High-risk patients" refers here to those patients who have incurable diseases and those who have conditions which make them likely candidates for sudden and unexpected deaths. The statement that hospitals differed in actual numbers of death *was assumed* from the students' reported experiences. No effort was made to confirm or deny these impressions by obtaining the actual death statistics from the hospitals in question.

In no school was there centralized planning for assignments to dying patients, with two significant results. In general, the students encountered death and dying on a chance basis. The outcomes for the students—whether positive, neutral, or traumatic—depended on the combination of circumstances surrounding each incident or series of incidents. At the opposite extreme, some students completed school without witnessing death and without participation in the care of a person in the final stages of illness. The assignment purpose played a major part in effecting these results.

Assignment Purpose

In all of the schools the use of patient assignments was influenced by an amalgamation of two different ideologies—the traditional hospital-work orientation and the newer psychiatric emphasis on nurse-patient relationships and communication skills. In the schools administered by hospitals the former ideology was predominant, whereas the university school was strongly imbued with a psychiatric focus on patient care. Patient assignments in all the schools were similar during the first six months. However, what the teachers felt was important determined not only the kinds of nursing techniques the students practiced but also what the students came to feel was important.[8]

In reading the remainder of this chapter, one should be aware that the differences between the teaching programs in the university school and in the hospital schools could not be classified strictly by types of schools. Rather, the variations in assignment patterning appeared as differences in degree rather than kind.

[8] In a study entitled "Satisfying and Stressful Situations in Basic Programs in Nursing Education," Fox and Diamond and their associates found that student descriptions of patient care covered four main categories—administering physical care, administering emotional care, recovery or death of a patient, and relationships with the patient. David J. Fox and Lorraine K. Diamond, in association with Ruth C. Walsh and Lucille Knopf, *Satisfying and Stressful Situations in Basic Programs in Nursing Education* (New York: Columbia Teachers College, 1964).

There were some major differences, to be sure. The heavy emphasis placed on the interpersonal aspects of nursing by teachers in the baccalaureate program caused these students to become acutely sensitive to the emotional needs of patients and thereby led some of the students into assignment difficulties not generally encountered by students in the other programs. In varying degrees of intensity, however, the programs in the hospital schools also gave attention to teaching about the psychological care of patients. Also important, some of these schools were altering their assignment practices so that they more closely resembled the laboratory pattern used by the faculty in the university school. No doubt these changes were causing the students to undergo experiences not unlike those encountered by students in the baccalaureate program. The discussion which follows is written to show a clear distinction between the results for students when different assignment contexts are used. A direct comparison of the schools among themselves was not done. The assignment policies employed by the five schools are listed in Appendix B and can be used to assess the similarities and differences of the assignment contexts provided by them.

Within the university school, patient assignments were defined as laboratory practice, with the hospital as only one of many practice fields. The patient assignment was an integral part of each nursing course, and the intent was to provide practice in solving problems associated with a specific area of nursing practice.[9] The curriculum emphasized the importance of nurse-patient interaction, and laboratory practice within the nursing courses was structured to maximize the opportunity for students to talk with patients and sometimes with their families as well.

During the first year the time allotted to laboratory practice was limited to nine hours weekly, thereby restricting the time and opportunity for students to practice giving direct care to their assigned patients. Also the stress given to the interpersonal aspects of nursing meant that less attention was devoted to gaining skill

[9] The four areas were medical-surgical nursing, maternal and child nursing, psychiatric nursing, and community health nursing.

in performing physical procedures and manual techniques. One important and far-reaching effect was that some students were assigned to give nursing care to critically ill patients when they were so unsure of themselves that they became immobilized by the assignment. A student who had such an experience during her first year made this observation.

> I just remember feeling so helpless and not knowing. I did not know what to do, yet I knew that there had to be something that could have been done, but I was just standing there watching him die. I think this hit me hardest of all, just to stand there and look at him as if he were a guinea pig. I remember just going into the room, picking up objects and moving them around. The wife and son were standing there trying to talk with him but he just seemed so much in a coma that he wasn't paying attention to them. I remember walking out of the room and going into the utility room and repeating things over and over again just more or less to get out of the room.

A student experience of this sort was likely to occur when the teacher who selected the assignment was inexperienced as a teacher, and also new in the school. It was also likely to happen when a curriculum was in transition and new approaches to teaching were being tried. Program innovation was not limited to the university school. In fact, one of the hospital schools was initiating extensive curriculum change while the data for this study were being collected.

The patient assignment was utilized somewhat differently when the principal objective was practice in performing traditional hospital tasks. When the latter ideology predominated in a school, the course in fundamentals of nursing emphasized physical and technical nursing care. Patient assignments were chosen primarily to provide opportunities to practice these techniques. Each student was assigned to one or two patients for short periods of time (usually three to four hours, twice a week), and the teachers supervised their activities closely. The teaching practice of close supervision of student performance was used in all of the schools during the first semester that students were assigned to give direct care to hospitalized patients.

Once the course in fundamentals was completed, the use of patients more clearly demonstrated the basic ideology of the school. An orientation toward hospital work generally resulted in a decrease in direct supervision, combined with an increase in assignment expectations. In one school, for example, the students changed from having practice periods of three hours to work days of eight hours—including weekends. At the same time the assignment load increased from one and two patients to four and five. Although the teachers were responsible for selecting these patients in accordance with course requirements, the teachers were not always present when the students needed help in performing assigned tasks. Thus the students increasingly relied on the staff nurses for advice and assistance. On the weekends patient assignments were made by the hospital nursing staff, and the instructors were seldom around to check on these assignments.

During the summer, assignment to the hospital wards was continued in schools which had short vacation periods. During these weeks the students functioned essentially as members of the hospital staff because the instructors were seldom available, or at best, only a skeleton instructional staff was at work. In the other schools the students could work in the hospital for pay during the summer, and sometimes during the regular school year as well. In fact, students in all of the schools had opportunities to encounter death while not under the direct supervision and guidance of the teaching staff.

In the hospital schools direct supervision by teachers decreased —usually after the first year. At the same time, the school assignment became similar to a regular hospital work assignment. Sometimes there were few safeguards to protect the student from a "bad experience." For example, a student could have a difficult encounter with a dying patient before she had had sufficient experience to feel sure of herself as a nurse under ordinary working conditions. One student told about an assignment to a patient who had attempted suicide.

This lady was admitted with puncture wounds of her abdomen and it was rather a hurried situation. When I was asked to go into the room to help, I didn't know it was a suicide. I didn't know anything about it except that I was needed to help. I went in and I did sort of assume that she had an accident, or something. She was covered with blood from her shoulders to about her knees. I couldn't at the time see the puncture wounds. The intern at the time told me to stay with her and not to leave the room under any circumstances, and it didn't dawn on me why. I was taking her blood pressure, and I was trying to clean her up a bit. I was told that a special nurse had been called, and I was just trying to get as much cleaned up before she arrived. I did have to leave the room for a brief moment at one time, and that was when I found out that the doctor had said that I should not leave because it was a suicide attempt. I just walked out the door, and that was how I found out. So I went back in and stayed there as if I were a dumb statue on the side of the bed.

The hospital work assignment can be extremely hazardous for a student when she is assigned to the ward during a period of heavy work pressures because the chance of making a performance error increases under these conditions. One student described the following experience.

I'll tell you about one horrible mistake I made, which I can talk about now, but I almost left school I was so upset about it. I was working on the same ward where I am now, and we had quite a full house, and there was an RN coming into the ward, and we had a couple of students and aides and orderlies working. It was rushed, and there were patients who were pretty sick. I'm rationalizing again, anyway, I had one patient who was in DT's, or on the verge of it. So I was going to give him some paraldehyde. Our solutions are in a locked cupboard for external use, I mean one for internal, and it is clearly labeled. I very nicely used formaldehyde instead of paraldehyde, can you imagine. Luckily, it was discovered. I don't know what I would have done if it wasn't discovered. That patient was taken to emergency and his stomach was pumped out. It was quite a learning experience.

Thus the use of evening and night shifts, particularly on busy wards and without supervision, increases the probability of a traumatic incident, because the student carries great personal responsibility under conditions which are conducive to the use of imprecise habits of working. Giving the wrong medicine is far easier to do when one is assigned to a busy ward alone than when under the direction of a teacher. One might also speculate about the errors unknowingly committed under these conditions.

Under assignment conditions of this nature, the student must often decide how to deal with many kinds of patient problems, including unexpected deaths and patients who "take forever" to die. When faced with assignments which required decisions about these problems, the students learned many of the tactics used by practicing nurses for controlling themselves and for minimizing personal involvement with patients and families.[10] They also picked up some of the ways used by seasoned hospital nurses for managing death and dying as work problems. On the night shift, for example, the nurses might make every effort to keep a patient alive until the change of shift to avoid the tedious and time-consuming task of postmortem care. Some students learned this practice of "riding patients out."

In the hospital schools, the selection of patients was sometimes delegated by the teachers to the hospital staff. Under these circumstances assignments were likely to be made principally to take care of the work needs on the wards. Less attention was given to the students' needs to learn. A student commented about these assignments in this way.

> The faculty always try to give us patients that have something that we have been recently studying, if it's possible. On the weekends, we are on our own. We usually get more patients, and we don't give medications on the weekends because the instructor is not around. We can get anything on the weekend. It seems to me that we have more work to do. They give us

10 See Glaser and Strauss, *op. cit.*, pp. 226–256, for a discussion of the development and use of strategies for maintaining composure when faced with caring for dying patients.

four or five patients or six without qualms because the nurses feel that they won't have the instructors around their necks.

Some students described themselves as being assigned to more than their share of critically ill and difficult patients. Others recalled the significant impressions left when they encountered several patient deaths in succession. As a consequence of their experiences with the hospital work assignment, at the end of three years some students had developed a sharp distaste for hospital work. One senior made this comment.

> One of the doctors recently asked me to work for him after graduation, and I would like an office job. He asked me why I felt this way, and I told him I'm tired of all the running around we do. I think you get emotionally involved in the hospital, and I think I do need a change.

In the university program, selection of patients and clinical supervision were controlled by the faculty and infrequently delegated to the hospital nursing staff. There were, of course, different interpretations of how best to implement this teaching policy—thus some teachers were readily available to the students on the hospital wards, whereas others put in an appearance less frequently. Assignments were generally made for daytime hours. Only rarely did a teacher make assignments during the evenings. (Of course, this did not prevent the students from seeing their patients during these hours—often to collect the "basic data" required for their written assignments.) In general, the assignment practices protected the students from many of the work pressures of hospital life. Assignments to specific wards were generally short—usually two to four weeks, for eighteen to twenty-four hours weekly, and the patients chosen were seldom those in the final stages of illness. The attention given to death and dying by those engaged in clinical teaching was sporadic rather than routine, except for an emphasis on "grief work" by those teaching maternal–child nursing. A high proportion of students did not have assignments to dying patients, or did not recognize their patients as dying. The probability was high that a student could complete school with little or no experience in learning how to provide care for dying patients and their families.[11]

Within each school the assignment purpose significantly affected the likelihood and the conditions of student encounters with dying patients. However, the student perspective on care of dying patients was also influenced by the condition of accountability. To be accountable means to be called to explain one's conduct. The students were expected to give "causes and effects" for many of their actions to several different authorities, the most powerful being their teachers. As students, their actions were governed by various rules and constraints—both explicit and implicit —imposed by the culture of the school and the culture of the hospital. During the socialization process the students learned to give importance to those matters for which they were held responsible by their teachers and by their own version of the nursing culture.[12]

Accountability, as Student and as Nurse

When nurse students are assigned to provide nursing care for patients, they are responsible on two levels—as students and as nurses. The assignment to a critically ill patient may be not only a test of one's performance as a safe and adequate nurse, but also a test of one's progress as a student in school. As a school assignment, the patient assignment *must* be completed according to the

[11] What these data had suggested was supported by data from another study. Fifty per cent of the class (total N of 38) who were in the baccalaureate program and graduated in 1963 had not witnessed the death of a patient to whom the individual student had been assigned. Twenty-nine per cent reported that they had not had the experience of dealing with the family of a dying patient. These data were provided by the Nursing Careers Project (USPHS Grant NU 00024), School of Nursing, University of California, San Francisco Medical Center. Staff members: Fred Davis, Virginia Oleson, Elvi Whittaker.

[12] In a study of medical students, the student perspective on clinical practice was observed to be strongly governed by ideas of *medical responsibility and experience*. See Howard S. Becker, et al., *Boys in White* (Chicago: University of Chicago Press, 1961), pp. 221–238.

teacher's expectations. In addition, there are other school requirements to be met. The student is responsible for satisfactory completion of written reports and examinations and for appropriate
participation in class discussions. The student is held accountable
for those things, the teacher considers to be important, and the
student estimates her progress from the cues given by test questions, grades, and clinical evaluation summaries. Put another way,
the student's actions are governed by the demands and constraints
of the school's environment—or, more precisely stated, by her
interpretation of these regulations.

The student perspective on what is important for the nurse in
the care of dying patients is directly related to what is emphasized
as important by their teachers. A low priority is attached to the
care of dying patients—those who have no possibility of recovery.
As one student put it "I knew that everything that I did on him
took time away from my other patient, who is going to be living
and has a good prognosis." A high value is associated with life-
saving actions and recovery activities.

> I would much rather be in on the beginning end of things. I
> would much rather be the nurse with a diabetic whose diag-
> nosis has just been discovered and is referred for follow-up than
> to get the diabetic who is in a coma and badly controlled. I
> would much rather be in on the preventive teaching end of it
> than to get the kiddies when they are good and sick, or anyone
> for that matter. It is just too depressing and too upsetting to
> me.

Specifically, the students tend to view death according to those
aspects of nursing practice for which the rules of conduct are
most explicitly defined, both by their teachers and by hospital
routines, and about which they must usually report back. The
student perspective on nurse responsibility with respect to dying
patients centers principally around the procedural and technical
activities associated with life-saving actions and with terminal care,
activities performed when there is no possibility of recovery. The
students readily assimilate the values, beliefs, and practices of the
nursing and the hospital cultures.

The teachers play a major part in influencing the students' perspective on what it means to be a nurse. They also play a major part in influencing the students' perspective on what it means to be a student. In fact, they hold positions which permit them to decide whether or not a student can continue to be a student. Not surprisingly, the students are concerned about avoiding actions for which serious penalties can be invoked. A teacher's judgment of "unsatisfactory performance" carries a serious threat because the student who receives such an evaluation may be asked to withdraw from school. Within the accountability framework, the student perspective on the patient assignment is governed by three principal ideas: getting experience, pleasing the teacher, and avoiding negligent performance as a nurse.

From the student viewpoint, one important function of the patient assignment is to provide experience in performing nursing tasks so as to prevent the possibility of making mistakes in the future. One student stated her expectations in this way.

> As a student I learn things every day. As a student, you don't know when to recognize real dangers and when not to recognize them. It's hard to know which signs and symptoms are really significant. This is one area in which I feel insecure as a nurse.

In the student's eyes the patient assignment was valuable if it provided "good experience" in learning to do the technical tasks associated with patient care.

The student perspective on the patient assignment was greatly influenced by the growing importance given to the interpersonal aspects of patient care by nursing instructors. In all of the schools the teachers talked about the importance of psychological care. In the university school the amount of attention devoted to teaching this aspect of nursing practice was very high. Specific teaching techniques were used to stimulate the students to focus attention on their own behaviors, as well as on the behaviors of their patients. Very frequently the process recording became a fundamental instructional method for directing the student to look at her own feelings and actions.[13] The teachers frequently used the ward conference as a forum in which the students were expected to discuss their reactions to their assignments. Some teachers used individual conferences with the students for the same purpose, and these conferences were often scheduled on a weekly basis.[14]

Because of the intense focus on human reactions and on communication skills, some students at the university school became acutely sensitive to the emotional aspects of patient care. In their efforts to provide psychological care these students tended to get themselves into conversational dilemmas with their patients. The students often found themselves engaged in interactions in which they "should be able to do something," but they did not know what to do. One student said,

> She had a very strong faith, but she kept saying that she knew God meant this operation to be. Of course, she had a choice in having this or not; yet she knew that she would come out of it all right. She had had a master's student, and she would always bring this in. This made me a little nervous, simply because I didn't know how to support her in her religious beliefs because my background was such that I hadn't anyone as verbal. So I think this more than anything bothered me because

[13] Jeannette C. Nehren and Marjorie V. Batey, "The Process Recording: A Method of Teaching Interpersonal Relationships Skills," *Nursing Forum*, Vol. 2, No. 2 (1963), pp. 65–73. On page 66 these authors provide a definition of process recording, as follows, "the process recording is defined as the verbatim and seriatim recording, to the extent that memory will permit, of the verbal and non-verbal interaction that has occurred between the patient and the nurse (or nursing student). It includes: (1) the written record of the verbal and behavioral communication which occurred between the participants; (2) written comments identifying the feelings that were experienced and those that she infers were experienced by the patient; and (3) the nurse's written analysis and evaluation of the meaning of the interaction and the clues to the patient's needs."

[14] One teacher who used this teaching approach viewed the instructor-student relationship as analogous to the student-patient relationship. See Margaret Wallace, "The Student and the Unwed Mother," *Nursing Forum*, Vol. 2, No. 2 (1963), p. 79.

she had kept saying that whatever happened was because God had wanted it to happen, and she knew that God wanted her to live through the operation.

Often the students left such assignments with feelings of guilt and inadequacy. A teacher reported a student's reactions in this way.

She said, this is one of the most startling things that she wrote, that she was aware many times during the morning that the patient was asking her for support, and that she (the student) could have given it to her. "But I didn't," as Mary (the student) phrases it, "I could have given it to her, but I did not. And I think this is the greatest mistake I made, and one which is unforgiveable, or should not be allowed to make," or something of that order.

Experiences of this sort were especially intense when the patient was known to be dying.

In spite of the emphasis given to psychological care, however, there were few teachers who offered guidance in how to talk with dying patients. The students became aware that many of their teachers were not prepared to offer them assistance with this problem. One student made this observation about a teacher.

It's funny, but I have the feeling that Miss Jones tried to talk openly about it, but yet I felt there was also the notion of let's just put it aside. Because so much emotion is involved, it seemed like she just didn't want to get in and unravel it. Just leave it alone, tie it up, and put it away in a corner.

The students learn that the rules governing the interactional aspects of nursing are more ambiguous than the regulations governing procedural and technical matters, and accountability to the teacher is subject to greater individual interpretation. Although judgments about student performance in providing physical care are generally made on the basis of direct observation, the teachers have to rely principally on indirect means in the form of verbal and written reports when judging interactional performance.

Teachers are not present when many student-patient conversations take place—thus the students can easily select the amount and kinds of information to report back to the teachers. The students learn rapidly that the social and psychological aspects of terminal care are not necessarily reportable.[15]

Only a few teachers at the university school held the students responsible for reporting back on their interpersonal contacts with dying patients. This approach was used primarily for teaching graduate students who were assigned to patients with chronic and long-term illness. These students did not have rotating assignments but carried one patient for prolonged periods of time. Their teachers emphasized the importance of nurse interactions with the patients and their families, rather than the traditional nursing tasks. The students were expected to report on their conversations by means of individual and group conferences and of written reports. Both the students and the teachers encountered many problems they had not anticipated. As they experimented with new ways of interacting with patients, families, physicians, and with each other, both the teachers and the students were engaged in redefining their roles as nurses.

A few teachers in the hospital schools used process recordings on something of a regular basis, usually in teaching pediatric or psychiatric nursing. Some instructors utilized ward conferences for talking with the students about their problems in planning and implementing their assignments to patients. With respect to the care of dying patients, one student observed,

> We have talked about the dying patient and terminal patients and the problems that they present. They feel the best way for us to do this is to talk in groups because it brings out—you're more apt to say something and contribute something in a group than you would alone.

---

[15] For a discussion of reportable and nonreportable actions relative to the care of dying patients in hospitals, see Anselm L. Strauss, Barney G. Glaser, and Jeanne C. Quint, "The Nonaccountability of Terminal Care," *Hospitals*, **38** (January 16, 1964), pp. 73–87.

These teaching practices—process recordings and psychologically focused conferences—were sporadic, however. In general, the students in the hospital schools learned to avoid interactions which might lead to emotionally disturbing results for them. They learned to give first priority to the technical problems associated with the care of dying patients.

In all schools the patient assignment is used under many different sets of conditions. Sometimes the student carries no responsibility as a nurse but enters the situation only as an observer. Sometimes she shares the responsibility with the teacher or with a staff nurse. On other occasions she may carry the equivalent of a hospital work assignment, with complete responsibility for patient welfare in her own hands. Under any of these conditions a student may perform ineptly or make an error in judgment, but the potential for a personally traumatic experience increases in proportion to the amount of direct nurse responsibility which the student carries by herself.

The importance attached by nurse teachers to life-saving and recovery goals made fear about negligent nurse performance a primary concern. No student wanted to make a serious mistake or perform in a way which might injure a patient. A sense of personal responsibility as a nurse is a major influence in the nurse student's judgment of her own actions. How she reacts depends not only on whether she *has* specific responsibility as nurse but, perhaps more important, whether she *sees herself as having* responsibility.[16] There are three conditions which maximize the possibility of actual or perceived negligent performance by a student: assignment to a new and unfamiliar setting, limited prior experience with the nursing problems to be solved, and little or no direct supervision or guidance by an experienced nurse.

For the nurse student, accountability *as a nurse* is a complicated matter because she is responsible to many different authori-

16 A nurse student can be negligent in fact by committing an illegal act or omitting one which has been judged by the law to be required under the particular circumstances. However, the student can also define herself as negligent if she fails to come up to her own expectations about "proper" performance in solving a given problem.

ties during the implementation of the patient assignment. A troublesome problem occurs when students find themselves responsible for implementing different sets of standards governing acceptable nursing performance. In all of the schools the students were aware of discrepancies between what their teachers taught was good nursing practice and what they saw being practiced by nurses on the hospital wards. In the hospital schools the students were sometimes caught directly between conflicting sets of instructions because they were held accountable both by their teachers and by the hospital staff. The students had to decide which persons were "right" and to act according to that choice. Criticism from either authority made a difficult assignment even more difficult, and even traumatic if the student considered the criticism unwarranted.

When the assignment involved a dying patient, the student was usually extremely sensitive to criticism, whether conflicting standards were involved or not. Thus one student described being terribly upset by the comments of a head nurse whom she had respected a great deal. In her words,

> I went back up to the floor to see him every day. I wasn't in anybody's way and wasn't cutting my own work time to go up there. He couldn't really talk to me because he was in a coma but I'm sure he knew that I was there, so I talked to him. It upset me very much when one of the head nurses whom I worked with really closely said, "Okay you, don't get involved!" I wasn't crying and being a big baby about the situation, but I really liked this patient. He was a good friend. He didn't have a family, and it was depressing to me to see how we'd worked and worked with him for four weeks. It kind of upset me to see this reaction by the nurses on the floor, and I almost felt like saying, "Well, we're still students." It was very unfair.

By their actions and comments the nurses on the wards can add to the difficulty of a student's assignment or, conversely, can make it easier for her. In commenting about her reactions to the preceding incident, the student continued,

I think I felt closer to this patient than with any other patient who has died, and I knew he was going to die. I didn't really cry, I mean it wasn't that it was a great loss. I think I cried mostly because of what the nurses had said because that's very depressing to me. After all, nurses are human too. We're taught to accept any individual as to how they react in a situation. This is the way I felt about this man, and yet it didn't seem to matter. *Supposed to act like a hard-working nurse, you know.*

Through experiences such as these, the students learn that composure and self-control are highly valued characteristics for the nurse. They also learn that those who violate the norms of the hospital and nursing cultures must suffer certain consequences.

When working relationships between the teacher and the ward staff are positive, the consequences for students are likely to be positive. Under these conditions the hospital nurses tend to be supportive, rather than critical, when the students come to them for assistance. If relationships between teacher and staff are strained or unclear, the students are likely to suffer the consequences—sometimes through direct criticism from the staff nurses. Because the teachers generally must rely on the ward nurses for information about the patients used as assignments, the nurses can also "take out their anger" by seeing to it that the students are assigned to difficult patients. The student can easily become a scapegoat when unresolved tensions among the teachers and the hospital staff are present in large numbers.

If only because it is carried out in a context in which students are accountable to multiple authorities, the patient assignment is a hazardous enterprise. Because of the high values accorded to life-saving actions by doctors and nurses, the assignment in which a patient dies is an especially hazardous enterprise for the student. A student's ability to meet an encounter with death in a responsible way—as a nurse and as a student—is very much affected by the accountability context in which the incident takes place.

When the assignment is such that the student shares responsibility as a nurse with other nurses, the chances are decreased that the student will have a traumatic encounter with death. For some students first encounters with death take place during the summer of the first school year while they are working closely with the hospital staff rather than with their teachers. Under these conditions the students have direct access to seasoned hospital workers, who offer them advance warning about hazardous patient assignments and help them live through the emotionally disturbing reactions which often accompany these first-time experiences, "I was lucky. I had two really good people with me that night. They helped me throughout, and I learned an awful lot." When a student encounters death under conditions of teamwork, such as these, she has access to support and encouragement, and the chances are high that she will have a positive experience. She can turn directly to another person for help in making decisions. She does not carry complete responsibility for what happens to the patient.

Sometimes the student looks to the nursing staff for guidelines in knowing what to say or do when an assignment is troublesome.

> Because the baby wasn't breathing properly at all, the mother was calling out, "Will it be all right?" They put her under, but the nurses all—I mean, the father was walking down the hall, pacing around, asking what it was. One nurse was avoiding him, and this bothered me a lot because nothing could make him more apprehensive, you know, unless there was something the matter. Yet as a decision, I didn't know what to do, and I don't know that I would know what to do right now as to what to tell him. So I stayed in the nursery because I felt I was safer. I didn't want to go out there and be confronted by him. I thought he could handle it better through the doctor.

As this incident implies, the nurses may not be able to provide direction for the student because they probably "don't know what to do" either. As a result, the student learns to move away from potentially disturbing interactions in the same way as do the nurses she observes on the hospital wards. Incidents involving the death of a patient often contribute to this kind of learning because many interactional activities associated with death in the hospital are not necessarily reportable to one's superiors, thus are outside of the accountability system.[17]

Sometimes a student can be in a patient situation in which she has little responsibility, either as a student or as a nurse. Then she is unlikely to feel inadequate or negligent on either score. At the other extreme, she can have an assignment which requires that she give a satisfactory accounting of herself both *as a nurse* and *as a student*. Under conditions of two-fold accountability, the student is doubly vulnerable to feelings of negligence should she make a mistake or be unable to function adequately.

> The doctor's orders were to give good terminal care. I didn't seem to be able to function at all that morning, even enough to give her a decent bed bath or to turn her as often as was ordered. She had labored breathing, she was catheterized, she had a rectal tube and oxygen and IV's. And this whole thing about keeping a patient alive when they really feel that there is no hope. It's terminal care, and you have all of these intravenous feedings and oxygen in attempts to keep her going. To me it just seemed that dying in itself was enough for the family, and then to be put into a situation to care for her, when I had never taken care of a seriously ill patient. I didn't feel that I got any support at all from my instructor, more of it was constructive criticism or not-so-constructive as to where I couldn't function, and I had better think about this, and look into it, which I knew. I needed someone to tell me this, I needed someone to talk to me, and to let me get my feelings out because I had nightmares while I took care of her, and I couldn't function very effectively.

If she performs well in both roles, of course, the chances are high that she will have a highly satisfactory and satisfying personal experience.

> It completely exposed me to just numerous aspects that the nurse would have to deal with. It has been a maturation process for me. I never realized what I had in me. I never thought

17 Strauss, Glaser, and Quint, *op. cit.*, p. 74.

that I would ever be able to cope with so many problems, and especially the baby's unexpected condition.

Whenever such an assignment involves a student's behavior in coping with death or dying, it carries a tremendous emotional impact—thus is likely to be remembered as a moment of terrible failure, or a moment of great success.

In Summary

This chapter has considered some of the organizational and ideological conditions which play a major part in determining what nurse students are taught about the care of dying patients. The student perspective on the care of dying patients reflects the basic values of nursing culture—a high priority is attached to the life-saving goals of practice. The students tend to define the nurse's role with dying patients primarily in terms of terminal-care procedures and activities performed at the time of death. Teaching practices which emphasize responsible behavior and avoidance of errors in practice cause the students to have high concerns about personal negligence. When the curriculum places a heavy emphasis on the importance of psychological care of patients, the students can also "feel negligent" during interactions which go awry. When these are with patients known to be dying, the students are likely to feel especially inadequate. The student perspective on dying patients is directly influenced by the content emphasized in the curriculum.

The probability that students will or will not be assigned to dying patients is a function of the assignment context developed by the school. The extent to which dying patients *are available* for assignment purposes is determined by the hospital locales utilized for practice. The extent to which the students actually encounter death is more directly a function of the purpose underlying the use of patients as school assignments. When the patient assignment as laboratory practice pattern is used without centralized planning for assignments to dying patients, the chances are high that students can complete school without this experience. When the hospital work assignment pattern is used without centralized planning for assignments to dying patients, the chances are high that students can encounter death under a wide variety of circumstances. Sometimes these encounters lead to very positive results, but often they do not.

Under either assignment pattern the students can have very positive experiences during assignments to dying patients. Under either assignment pattern the students can also have overwhelming assignments which leave them feeling terribly inadequate. The most critical condition affecting the results of patient assignments is the accountability factor that is present. Encounters with death are hazardous enterprises for students under the best of circumstances, when the student carries minimal responsibility as a nurse and she gets direction and support from an experienced person during the assignment. Paradoxically, the most positive and the most negative experiences for students take place under conditions of dual responsibility, when the student is held accountable both as a nurse and as a student. When these extreme experiences take place during encounters with death, they are usually turning points in the lives of the students. The students' views of themselves *as nurses*, and also as students, are strongly affected by critically important experiences in which they define themselves as successes or failures. The next chapter considers how the nurse teacher's perspective on death and on teaching influences what happens to students during these critical experiences—and also during other assignments in which dying patients are involved.

Chapter 3 | Teacher Perspectives on Death

The teacher's perspective on death is a powerful influence on her actions as nurse and as teacher. Either directly or indirectly she strongly affects what happens to students when they encounter dying patients on the hospital wards. The teacher's perspective on death most clearly manifests itself in her clinical teaching practices. In this regard three different teacher perspectives were observed to be important—the inexperienced teacher, the unaware teacher, and the concerned teacher. The teacher's perspective on death, however, is only one part of her perspective as a teacher. There are many other forces which shape her world of work and influence her ability to perform both as a nurse and as a teacher of nurses.

Conditions Affecting the Teacher's Work World

Whether she teaches in a college or in a hospital school, the nurse teacher in the 1960's lives in a markedly different work world than did her counterpart of twenty-five years ago. It is a world marked by change and unrest, with many different kinds of pressures—some of which have come into being (or have increased in severity) since the Second World War. There are several conditions which play a critical part in affecting the nurse teacher's view of her world and which influence how she chooses to function within it.

Rapid Changes in Medical Technology

The expansion of medical technology since 1945 has greatly influenced the practice of nursing. Scientific developments have contributed to tremendous changes in the functions of hospitals, where the majority of nurses are employed.[1] In many of these institutions diagnostic and therapeutic techniques have increased both in complexity and in number. Both medical and nursing practices are undergoing changes to meet the demands imposed by these new procedures.[2] Correspondingly, for the teacher of nurses, expansion of medical knowledge has affected the content of nursing courses. The question of what to teach is no simple matter when knowledge is accumulating at so rapid a rate, yet this question must constantly be faced and answered in some way by those responsible for developing nursing courses. Not only does the knowledge explosion pose problems for broad curriculum planning, it also poses problems for the individual teacher who must decide how to keep pace with changes in her own field of specialization.

Changing Relationships Between Medicine and Nursing

As medical technology has expanded, both medicine and nursing have undergone fragmentation—with increased numbers of specialty workers involved in providing medical and nursing ser-

[1] According to American Nurses' Association, *Facts About Nursing, 1964 Edition* (New York: American Nurses' Association, 1964), p. 18, more than 63 per cent of all nurses are employed in hospitals.
[2] Cecil G. Sheps and Miriam E. Bachar, "Changing Patterns of Practice—Nursing and Medical," *North Carolina Medical Journal*, 25 (October, 1964), pp. 435–438.

vices within the hospital. With this change in the numbers of persons involved, open communication between doctors and nurses has become increasingly difficult to maintain. Misunderstanding between the two groups has grown.[3] During this same period schools of nursing have initiated curriculum changes which have minimized participation by physicians in the teaching of nurses. There has been a decreased use of physicians as lecturers, with more teaching responsibility assumed by nurses. Also, because the students spend less time on the hospital wards than in the days when they staffed the hospitals, the doctors have fewer opportunities to work with them directly. In their efforts to upgrade and improve the teaching of nurses, nurse educators have unwittingly alienated many physicians by excluding them from a dominant part (which they formerly held) in the instruction of nurse students.

The separation of nursing education and nursing service has also fostered a separation between nurse teachers and physicians. The teachers, in general, have no real responsibility for patient care in the hospital.[4] Because the teachers are concerned with school activities rather than with hospital activities, they have few personal contacts with physicians—except to discuss a teaching problem. Under these conditions the doctor has limited opportunities to see the nurse teacher either practicing nursing herself or effecting changes in practice through working with the ward nurses. Although some nurse teachers do present a favorable picture of themselves as practitioners, the working conditions prescribed by the school of nursing do not always make this move possible. Also, not all teachers see the necessity for assuming such a role. One outcome of this separation between medicine and

[3] A perceptive discussion of some of the roots of this misunderstanding is given by Edmund D. Pellegrino in "The Communication Crisis in Nursing and Medical Education," *Nursing Forum*, Vol. 5, No. 1 (1966), pp. 45–53.

[4] David Fox, et al., "Characteristics of Basic Nursing Faculty," *Nursing Outlook*, 12 (December, 1964), p. 41, points out that 88 per cent of the faculty appointments in twenty-three schools of nursing (eighteen were diploma schools) had no nursing service responsibilities.

nursing education has been an open expression of criticism by many physicians toward what is happening in schools of nursing. When highly critical comments are directed toward students and teachers in the ward setting where students are assigned for practice, a mood of uncertainty and conflict can easily be created. A work environment in which dissension predominates can add further to the strain of the nurse teacher's daily work.

Changing Relationships Within Nursing

It is not just with physicians that nurse educators sometimes find themselves in disagreement. The separation of nursing education and nursing service—initiated for the justifiable purpose of getting nursing schools on a sound educational basis—has created a disunity between nurses who teach and nurses who practice, particularly in hospitals. Part of this gap in understanding came about because the supervisors and head nurses, like the physicians, were excluded from much responsibility for teaching students. Thus the service staff found themselves with no tangible identification with the school or its policies. Smith has suggested that this disunity goes deeper than the usual conflicts and disagreements observed between the realists (the practitioners) and the idealists (the educators) of any profession because of a general failure on the part of nurses to identify with nursing as a profession. In her view the disunity seems to have resulted in nursing "getting its cues for action (in practice, education, and research) from physicians, hospitals, educators, social scientists, and others rather than from the society it purports to serve." [5]

Meyer suggests that there is a sharp discontinuity between the nurse's image of nursing, as projected by the nurse educator, and the actualities of her work life. The student meets the rough impact of reality on her first job.[6] When students are exposed to an educational philosophy of personalized patient care, they become highly critical of the performance of regular staff nurses and

[5] Dorothy M. Smith, "Education and Service Under One Administration," *Nursing Outlook*, 13 (February, 1965), p. 55.

[6] Ralph H. Meyer, "Professional Status of Nursing," *Hospital Topics*, 42 (May, 1964), pp. 35–39.

progressively disenchanted with the hospital as a projected work area.[7] A broad discrepancy exists between the projected ideal of the bedside nurse giving highly individualized care and the reality of hospital work—often routinized and impersonal. The difference in viewpoint of the teacher and the practitioner can lead to communication difficulties which prevent them from working together effectively.

There is another important basis for difference, sometimes conflict, between the instructor and the hospital nurses. Because the former does not carry direct responsibility for patient care, she is an outsider. As such, she may not show appreciation for the specific pressures of hospital work and for the difficult decisions faced by the ward nurses. She often is on the wards for short periods of time. She may be openly critical of what she sees being done. Viewed often as a threat, she must negotiate with the staff to establish a mutually satisfactory working relationship, without which there can be difficulties for her, and often for the students as well. If strain and tension exist, the teacher may well be blocked from obtaining information which can have an important effect on a student's assignment. For example, the instructor may give the student an erroneous picture of what is happening because she lacks certain facts. One teacher told a student that a newborn, not yet seen by his mother, would be taken out to the mother when all of the babies went out. When this event did not take place, the student became very upset. Only then did the teacher learn that a nerve injury had occurred during delivery and the doctors had not yet told the mother about it.

Sometimes instructors must teach on more than one ward, or be assigned to unfamiliar clinical settings. In the latter instance, they may face the added problem of feeling inadequate as nurses because they lack experience with the specific nursing problems found in that setting. One teacher spoke in retrospect about the effect of such an assignment on her ability to teach effectively,

[7] Fred Davis, Virginia L. Olesen, and Elvi Waik Whittaker, "Problems and Issues of Collegiate Nursing Education," in Fred Davis, ed., *The Nursing Profession* (New York: Wiley, 1966), pp. 138–175.

"I think that I made a mistake. I didn't prepare them adequately for doing this last year."

The Changing World of the Nurse Teacher

Perhaps the greatest pressure on the nurse teacher comes from the school itself and from the work demands prescribed by her position as a teacher. These demands are of two kinds—the specific responsibilities required by the school in which the teacher is employed, and the broader pressures exerted by a nationwide movement for improvement in nursing education. These demands are not mutually exclusive, of course, because changes brought about through such forces as the national accreditation program have had a profound effect on faculty responsibilities in individual schools. For one thing, the movement of nursing programs into colleges and universities has brought new types of pressures to bear on the nurse educator—for example, the university emphasis on research and publication as requirements for advancement.

There are several changes which have profoundly affected the daily activities of individual teachers in all schools of nursing. There has been an increased emphasis on the importance of clinical teaching, and on the teacher's responsibilities for selecting patients and for supervising students on the wards. This requirement is a time-consuming activity if the teacher is expected to be present on the wards whenever the students are there. Also it is not a simple task—particularly if students are in the first year—because the teacher must constantly decide which students to supervise directly, which can perform with minimal help, and how to tell the difference between these types of students.

Another pressure on the teacher's time comes from the increased emphasis on student learning—implemented through such activities as individual conferences, the use of process recordings, and written summaries of student progress. Schools of nursing have become more and more student oriented, and much of the teacher's time is now devoted to individual and small-group activities. Less time and attention are given to traditional classroom teaching. These pressures are greatest on teachers in collegiate nursing programs, but the influence of these ideas is gradually being felt by faculties in other schools of nursing as well.

Another important influence is the trend toward curriculum experimentation combined with an emphasis on patient-centered teaching. One effect associated with this movement has been a lessened emphasis on specialization and a heightening of the notion of the nurse generalist.[8] For the nurse teacher this shift has brought specific and sometimes difficult problems, for instance, having to supervise students in an unfamiliar specialty setting or being responsible for new class content. When the curriculum is based on the "generalist" concept of nursing practice, the teacher's responsibilities are often less clearly defined than in a school where teaching assignments are specialized and specifically spelled out. An element of uncertainty when responsibilities are not clearly defined can be a tension-producing factor—both for individual teachers and for the faculty as a whole.

The work world of the nurse teacher is marked by unrest and change, with a high proportion of time devoted to student-centered tasks. Many decisions about teaching, however, are not predetermined but are left to the judgment of the individual instructor. What is taught about death and the care of dying patients is determined to a great extent by each individual's perspective on the matter. Several conditions play an important part in the development of these individual perspectives. Perhaps the most important has to do with the teacher's prior experience with death.

Conditions Affecting Perspectives on Dying

The Impact of Personal Experience

The extent to which a nurse teacher is comfortable in teaching about nursing care involving the dying patient is greatly influenced by her own prior personal experience with death. The

[8] A discussion of the influence of this shift on the curricula of different schools is presented in Faye E. Abdellah *et al.*, *Patient-Centered Approaches to Nursing* (New York: Macmillan, 1961).

teachers who can openly talk with students about these matters are those who through personal experience have come face to face with their own concerns about dying, most commonly through the experience of a death in their own family. Among younger teachers there are a few who describe the positive importance of a critical patient encounter during their student days, under the guidance of an understanding instructor. One young teacher reported this incident.

> None of the medical regime seemed effective with her, and we could see that she was getting worse, and we were pretty concerned. I think when I got closest to this, I got upset with my own feelings about it and did go to someone that I knew, who could help me with my feelings. This was an instructor who was not, at that point, directly concerned with the care of patients and this kind of business. So she helped me with my feelings about several different matters; here was somebody my age, in the hospital, what I felt about the blame, and what I thought about death, and what I thought my role was, and what I wanted to do, and I was scared, and that who was going to do it anyway, and who should do it, and all of this we investigated. No decision, you know, but at least I knew how I felt about it, which I hadn't known before.

Many more teachers, however, are still struggling with the unpleasant memories of difficult and distressing assignments they themselves had as students. Others have memories of unsatisfactory work experiences as nurses. There are also those who never had the experience of encountering death, either as students or as practicing nurses. Many instructors are unable to teach about the care of dying patients, except in a stereotyped traditional framework, because they themselves have not learned how to cope with death and dying. Instead, they are anxious about these matters.

The Influence of Course Content and Specialization

A teacher's perspective on dying as a nursing problem is also directly related to her area of specialization. Often what is taught about death derives from a partisan view of the subject. Instructors of psychiatric nursing, for example, tend to stress the importance of watching patient behavior so as to prevent the possibility of suicide. Teachers of courses on the fundamentals of nursing tend to focus on specific nursing activities required before a patient's death and at the time it occurs.

Those who carry the burden of teaching about the care of dying patients are instructors of medical and surgical nursing. In these areas the course content is more directly focused on physical illness than are courses in other nursing specialties, and the hospital wards used for practice are those in which the students are most likely to have direct encounters with dying patients. Often, however, these teachers emphasize nursing actions in meeting a pair of basic problems, how to cope with emergencies and how to provide physical comfort. Not uncommonly they assign students to patients with fatal diagnoses purely for practice in performing certain procedures. One teacher, for example, liked to assign students to patients with colostomies to give them experience in helping patients learn to adjust to a major change. In her words,

> I don't talk about emotional aspects as a separate category, but I think we deal with it when we talk about how to handle this kind of situation—how one can give reassurance to patients by the way that you do something and by your attitude toward it.

This teacher stressed the importance of the nurse doing colostomy care in a matter-of-fact way so as to convey a feeling of reassurance to the patient. She was aware that the question of cancer and death was often a problem for the patients and for the students, but she expressed reservations about the appropriateness of talking openly with these patients about their feelings on the matter. Like many nurse teachers, this instructor emphasized the hopeful aspects of nursing care. She did not see that assignments to terminal patients as such offered much to students, because the assignments "were depressing."

Although much that is taught about the care of dying patients covers little that is new, there are indications that different ideas are now being introduced by some teachers. For example, one instructor in medical-surgical nursing described a course containing a section on family development and gerontology. Her teaching included a discussion of death as a part of the normal life process. In the baccalaureate nursing program the teachers of maternal–child nursing stressed the importance of psychological care, and they talked about the nurse's responsibilities for working with the parents of dying children. Although there were class discussions about these matters, these teachers seemed primarily concerned about the students' reactions to their assignments and not very able to offer concrete suggestions for coping with specific problems. One class discussion, for example, centered around the issue of helping a family grieve for a dying child, yet students did not necessarily recognize bereavement behavior when they encountered it on the pediatric ward. In describing her reactions to working with the family of a six-year-old with an inoperable brain tumor, one student noted that the mother was making a "good adjustment," but she didn't like the way the grandmother behaved. In her view,

> You know she would go buy these expensive gifts and bring them in to him. She was always doing this. Sometimes when he was sleeping, she would come up and stand by the glass window and just stand there and look at him. She really sort of irritated me.

The student did not identify the grandmother's behavior as a form of bereavement. These teachers were concerned about helping the students with a difficult nursing problem, but the guidelines they offered for working with a grieving family were often vague. Like many teachers who were interested in the interpersonal aspects of patient care, they offered a general approach. The "hows" of implementing it were unclear to many of the students.

The Clinical Setting

Another condition which influences the teacher's perspective is the setting to which she is assigned. If she teaches on a high-risk ward, such as the intensive-care unit or emergency room, she is likely to emphasize life-saving activities. On a cancer ward she may well focus on comfort care. In either case the teacher cannot completely avoid the problem of death because the students encounter it almost every day. In contrast, some teachers are assigned to wards on which death seldom occurs, and their teaching makes little mention of the topic. The unexpected death on such a setting can be an extremely difficult problem—both for an involved student and for the teacher.

The clinical setting can have other important influences on the teacher's perspective. If working relationships with the staff are positive, the teacher can enjoy a pleasant work experience. If they are tense, she may well find clinical teaching a difficult job. She may also find herself frustrated by her own feelings about the ward. In describing her reactions to a geriatric ward, one teacher made this observation.

> When I first went there and I saw all those sad old people sitting there all crunched down, with their hands in front of their faces, I felt like a small grain of sand in the midst of a huge beach, and I wondered what I could do to precipitate any kind of change.

Expectations as Nurse and as Teacher

The clinical setting determines to a great extent whether the teacher will have to deal with death frequently or infrequently. Her own ideas about what constitutes *the* important nursing actions will influence what she stresses in her clinical teaching. If she views nursing principally in terms of physical care and the implementation of delegated medical tasks, her selection of patient assignments and her supervision of students will focus on those aspects of care. If she views nursing primarily as an interpersonal relationship, she will be interested in the student's involvement with her patients more than in the performance of manual tasks. What the teacher chooses to observe and what she chooses to discuss with the student are mainly determined by these expectations, and her teaching about death—if done at all—will be no exception.

The teacher is also influenced by her sense of responsibility for the welfare and safety of the assigned patients. If this perspective dominates her clinical teaching, she may well devote much of her time to supervising students as they perform potentially dangerous procedures. Concern about patient welfare is a realistic concern, especially when students are inexperienced. This aspect of clinical teaching can be so time-consuming that the teacher has little opportunity for helping students with other aspects of their assignments.[9] One teacher described her frustrations in this way, "There is so much focus here on baths, treatments, routine. I want to help these kids focus on the interpersonal, and on working with people." Not all teachers are so frustrated, of course, and some view their clinical teaching responsibilities primarily in terms of preventing student errors.

The teacher's expectations about student performance are not based solely on what the students do as nurses. The teacher is also interested in how well they demonstrate what they have learned as students—through examinations, written assignments, and class participation. She stresses the subject matter she deems important, and the students are expected to report back on these matters. In general, those teachers who are recent graduates, particularly of baccalaureate programs, are inclined toward the human relations philosophy of nursing practice and teaching.[10] By comparison, many teachers who became nurses during an earlier era continue to emphasize medically oriented subject matter and traditional nursing tasks. The teacher's philosophy will show itself in the way she uses the patient assignment as a device for student learning and in her approach to clinical teaching.

Although nursing instructors are responsible for other aspects

[9] There is a basis in reality for this concern because nurse students can be held liable for negligence. See Helen Creighton, *Law Every Nurse Should Know* (Philadelphia: Saunders, 1957), pp. 46–47.

[10] S. Dale McLemore and Richard J. Hill, in "Role Change and Socialization in Nursing," *The Pacific Sociological Review*, 78 (Spring, 1965), pp. 21–27, found that recent nursing graduates were more "democratic" in their work orientations than were those who graduated at an earlier period. A similar finding was noted for nurses with a college degree in comparison with those without.

of the program, the emphasis here is on clinical teaching because it is in the direct encounter with dying patients that students most often run into difficulty. Some teachers are quite unaware of the impact of these encounters because their own perspective on dying is essentially one of avoidance. Others are prone to omit such assignments to protect the students, and probably themselves, from situations which might be terribly upsetting. Still others have unrealistic expectations about students' abilities to cope with these assignments—some anticipating expert performance and others anticipating students to "fall apart" in the situation.

The teacher's viewpoint on students, on assignments, and on death all contribute to what happens to the students when they encounter dying patients while under her direction. Three perspectives were found to be especially influential in these matters— the inexperienced teacher; the teacher who is unaware of the significance of these assignments; and the teacher who is concerned about helping students learn how to interact productively with dying patients. These perspectives do not appear in pure form in any one teacher, but rather can be thought of as themes which have different degrees of predominance in the viewpoints of all nurses who are engaged in clinical teaching.

Types of Perspectives

The Inexperienced Teacher

Historically, nursing has had something of a do-it-yourself approach to practice, and new teachers can find themselves in just this position with respect to clinical teaching. The new teacher may not have access to a seasoned instructor to assist her in making decisions, thus she learns by trial and error. The beginning teacher tends to *feel the pressure* of her responsibility for the students she is supervising. The strain can be intense if she has a large group of students, if her students are in their first year, or if she has had little work experience as a nurse.

Although this is not always true, the inexperienced teacher is likely to be assigned to a clinical setting which is unfamiliar. In addition to teaching *per se*, she has the important task of establishing work relationships with the staff—to facilitate the selection of patients and to ensure cooperation for herself. Work commitments within the school may limit her opportunities to have direct contacts with physicians—including the problem of trying to work closely with a rotating house staff. Thus she may find herself relatively isolated from the doctors and thereby deprived of useful information about what is happening to patients. If she has also had little personal experience with death and dying, she will be unprepared to recognize the meaning of certain events, and to forewarn the students about them.

The inexperienced teacher is a prime candidate for getting both herself and a student into a troublesome assignment involving a dying patient. She is new on the job and is unfamiliar with what is expected of her. If the curriculum is in transition, she may be quite unprepared for the problems she will meet, even though she has had prior teaching experience.[11] For instance, one teacher was surprised to find that students in their second year of school were manually inept. She was accustomed to students who were "taught how to do things." Like the beginning nurse student, the new instructor is prone to make errors in judgment because her previous experience has not always prepared her for the kinds of decisions she will have to make.

Like any nurse, the teacher can be upset if she makes a mistake which threatens to harm a patient. However, she can have the additional problem of appearing inadequate in the eyes of the student, and the ward nurses too, if she herself cannot cope with a specific nursing problem. She can also feel responsible for patient welfare if the student makes a mistake. The "guilt" can be even more severe if the teacher thinks she did not offer the student sufficient help. As a nurse she can feel responsible for the patient. As a teacher she can feel responsible for the student. She can also be concerned about other matters, such as criticism from

11 A teacher can be completely inexperienced (i.e., has never been a teacher) or can be relatively inexperienced (i.e., has not been a teacher in this school until recently but has taught elsewhere).

the hospital staff or her own adequacy as an instructor. In describing an upsetting incident which took place during her first year, one teacher made these comments about herself.

> I had lots of feeling myself because I had told her that I did not think he was going to die, and he did, which made me feel like a liar. I had used poor clinical judgment, and she had reacted with a great deal of feeling. I wanted to know whether I had pushed her into something that she couldn't handle or what I had done to her. She's a student who was not used to looking at her own reactions to herself, or to nursing or to anything. I was afraid for a little while that this was a pretty drastic mistake.

Not only did the instructor feel responsible for getting the student into the situation, she was afraid that the student might withdraw from nursing because of the experience.

The assignment became a significant experience for this teacher when the patient abruptly entered a critical state. The student was unable to stay in the room to complete the assignment because she was so upset by what had happened. The teacher questioned her own ability as a teacher in making the assignment, but she also wondered what the staff thought about the student's behavior. In her words,

> The graduates on the station—I wondered what their reaction would be to a student leaving an assignment. Many of these nurses came from programs like mine, where you sort of "do or die," and you don't run out on a patient. They seemed to have no negative feelings about her having done this, and I think were helpful to her.

She was relieved that the nurses had not passed judgment on the student, nor on *her* ability as a teacher. In retrospect, she thought that she might give the same assignment again, but, "I wouldn't have told her that he wasn't going to die."

Although this teacher was aware that the experience had been difficult for the student, she was far more intensely involved in her own fears and concerns as a teacher. She did not realize the tremendous impact the assignment carried, nor did she realize that the incident had become the talk of the class for several months afterward. Her lack of experience contributed to a traumatic experience, both for herself and for the student, chiefly because she was unaware that her actions could pave the way for such an occurrence. There are other teachers who are unaware of these possibilities, but not because of lack of experience as teachers.

The Unaware Teacher

The unaware teacher is one who is relatively "blind" to the impact of assignments to dying patients. Usually this teacher does not know what kinds of difficulties the students encounter during these assignments. For example, the students in one school frequently discussed the difficulties they had in talking with patients who were not to be told the diagnosis, yet one of their teachers was quite unaware that they had any problem. In her words, "I don't think so. I think that they are able to handle it. We talk about it, and they realize that the doctor has a reason for it. They accept it, and it doesn't seem to be a problem." Sometimes lack of awareness is directly related to conditions which prevent a teacher from being present when a crucial event takes place. Thus, her committee assignments may be such that she must delegate teaching responsibilities to others because these other school commitments take precedence. Not uncommonly, however, the teacher is unaware of the meaning of dying patient assignments because she is preoccupied with other matters: the safety of the patient, the students' learning of certain facts, or their professional behavior on the wards. An overconcern with such matters can sometimes block a teacher from recognizing the traumatic effects that a particular assignment may have for a student.

There are some teachers who have a personal need to avoid the subject of death because of their own discomfort when a patient is dying—sometimes because they had such terribly traumatic experiences with death when they were students. Not uncommonly such a teacher uses teaching practices which minimize her personal involvement with the topic and which protect her from direct contact with death and dying. She talks about the care of patients in generalities rather than specifics. As one teacher explained,

> I have not made a big topic of it. I have incorporated it as we talk about the different diseases. The girls have had terminal care in fundamentals, and then I talk about handling the patients in terminal situations and handling the family—how the patients react, family reactions, how they can help the family, a little bit about their own reactions to it.

She may not use terminal patients for assignments, or she may turn the entire matter of patient selection over to the ward staff. She tends to avoid direct supervision of the student and often does not know about recent experiences which the students have had. The unaware teacher may say that students have difficulties when faced with these assignments, but she is not aware of the specific problems they encounter or of the many traumatic episodes which take place.

Another kind of lack of awareness is demonstrated by the teacher who uses the dying patient assignment because the student "needs the experience." One teacher made this comment about a first-year assignment,

> I thought it would be good experience for her. I knew the patient was going to die. It seemed fairly certain she would die soon, but Mary had struck me as rather brittle, and I was trying to give her responsibility, and also to see if some of the brittleness might go. She's a very capable student as far as written work goes, understanding pathological physiology, but she has always been the first one to leave the ward—always the first one through. It makes you wonder how much warm rapport or feelings she actually has for the patient.

This type of assignment is made for a specific purpose other than care of the dying—usually care given the critically ill, or for practice in an emergency. Characteristic of the unaware teacher who uses this assignment pattern is her failure to recognize the frightening effect of these assignments when they are used before students are able to cope with them and her tendency to provide minimal direction and help during the assignments. In general, her lack of awareness derives from an unrealistic expectation about the student's ability to manage either the technical or the interactional aspects of a given patient assignment.

In a similar way there are teachers who have unrealistic expectations about the psychological components of patient care, and they make use of an assignment that is paradoxical because of its contradictory directives. They teach the students to encourage patients to explore and clarify their feelings while at the same time telling the students that they cannot mention the diagnosis until the doctor has discussed it with the patient. Too often, when the student encourages the patient to talk, he wants to talk about the very thing she has been told not to discuss. Thus the student finds herself in an impossible situation. As one student put it, "It's awful being expected to do something and not knowing how—and not being told how, or given help in doing this." Teachers who use this type of assignment appear to be unaware of the many stresses and strains provoked by its conflicting demands.

The Concerned Teacher

The concerned teacher is well aware of the specific difficulties students face in their contacts with dying patients, but she is not always certain about the best way to teach about this aspect of nursing care. Concerned teachers have one common characteristic. Through personal or professional experience they have come face to face with their own inadequacies in coping with many of the problems nurses face in providing care to dying patients, and they see a need for helping nurse students learn how to manage these assignments. One such teacher saw the difficulties students had in relating to patients with cancer and sought help for herself through weekly conferences with a medical social worker. In her words, "I just felt that I really needed help in solving my own problems in relating to this patient so that I could, in turn, help the student do the same." As a consequence, this teacher found herself better able to provide guidance for students when they encountered similar conversational difficulties.

Unlike many nurse teachers these instructors do not avoid talking about death, though they may have no answers to many questions which are raised. Rather than wait for the students, they often initiate conversation about these matters, either individually or in ward conferences. These teachers tend to recognize when students are extremely upset by certain patient assignments. They provide help either through direct assistance at the time or through discussion with the students later about the problems that were encountered.

Teachers with this perspective are concerned about helping students learn to work more effectively with dying patients, but they are often perplexed about what to do as teachers. They try different teaching approaches yet often wonder about the effectiveness of their actions. One teacher who utilized role playing to give students practice in talking with persons who persist in bringing up that crucial question—"Do I or don't I have cancer?"—was unsatisfied with the technique because, "I kept having the feeling that the only thing that happened was a lot of anxiety among the students." Another teacher wondered whether or not to pull students out of assignments when they became involved with the patients.

Although such teachers sincerely want to help students, they are hampered by two problems. They do not have well-formulated notions of what is involved either in helping a patient to die in his own way or in helping a student learn to do this. Also, they are unprepared for the kinds of reactions students have when they become involved in their own feelings about death and dying. One teacher who was working with graduate students in a course in cancer nursing made this observation about class discussions.

The second time I taught cancer nursing, the students didn't want to leave the topic of death for a long time. During that

long period of time one of the things I was not prepared for
was that one student actually grieved for a friend who had
died seven years before. She herself had never been permitted
and had not permitted herself to grieve. She had not been able
to talk about death as much as the rest of the class, but apparently she felt comfortable enough to grieve. This was almost
a whole class period. The other students were able to let her
go through this. She expressed great relief after. She had never
been able to do this and to see how it interfered with her
caring for patients. She'd placed certain barriers in the way of
expectations about how other people should behave. She didn't
think she had permitted other people to grieve either.

That this kind of teaching is difficult is demonstrated by the in-
stuctor's additional comment concerning this class. "It was terribly
uncomfortable because I kept thinking I don't know just how
far to go to be of help to her."

The concerned teacher is struggling to help the student develop a personalized approach to the care of dying patients, but
she is also struggling with defining her own role as teacher. Not
uncommonly she finds that this kind of teaching is an emotionally
strenuous experience for her as well as for the students. In part,
the tension exists because the teacher does not have clear guidelines for determining what her actions should be as both she and
her students become involved in their own feelings of helplessness
and hopelessness and frustration. One teacher made this observation about a given incident,

I felt a lot more feeling than I usually feel. I don't know if it
was because the student that I was so proud of was mad at
me, or if I had a real desire to help her—more than you usually do. I was more aware of really trying to get her to see
that she had done something and that this involvement was
not necessarily something to be avoided, or a negative thing,
as she was interpreting it when she came in for the conference.

Teachers of basic students were often well protected against the
consequences that pertain to dying patients because they were

caught up in teaching many other aspects of nursing practice. The teachers who were fully immersed in trying to cope with this difficult problem were those who were working with graduate students assigned to dying patients. By holding the students accountable for their interactions with patients who were facing death, these teachers found themselves engaged in a form of teaching which brought moments of great satisfaction, but also periods of tension and uncertainty and frustration.

Reactions to Teaching About Death

Nurse teachers may well minimize what they teach about the care of dying patients because the school of nursing is not organized to provide them with help in teaching about this difficult part of patient care. When individual teachers encounter specific problems in which death is a central concern, they usually must search for support informally, because the system does not have this kind of "backstopping" built into it. After an intense experience on the ward, one young teacher made this comment.

> I never felt a great booming lack of need, though there were times when I could have used some. I discussed the event rather casually, not in a guidance way, but by saying, "Thus and thus happened, and I have to talk to you about it." It was more like getting it off my chest, and telling a fellow faculty member what had happened.

The need for regular support is clearly expressed by instructors who are teaching students to interact more openly with dying patients. In one interview, the teacher's problem was defined in this way.

> The problem is helping students when they feel helpless. It's a difficult thing to hear people confess helplessness. What do you do about it? Probably at the times that we feel helpless in helping them, they're the most uncomfortable. It's like three levels of helplessness: the patient is helpless; the student is helpless; and I am feeling helpless.

To cope with such tensions, these teachers sought help on an *ad hoc* basis—usually from psychiatrists, social workers, and each other.

Teaching students new ways of interacting with dying patients is not easy teaching. The class sessions were usually centered on specific patient problems faced by the students.

> We usually focus on any patient that a student is taking care of, and they get *some* background information, not medical history, but an overview and attempt to identify what some of the problems are—whatever concerns the patient, what's happening with the communication in what they're doing. Some of them are doing process recording, so they read some of them, or selected portions of it.

Sometimes a teacher found herself becoming anxious because the "content" she thought was important did not always come up in class discussions.

> I don't know why really, because I think what we're doing and what we're learning is much more valuable than some of the things that we get anxious about, or worry about, or they can pick up by themselves very easily, in fact *are* in their readings.

Often these class discussions focused as much on the students as they did on the patients.

> The initial focus is on the patient, but it goes back and forth. I think as far as the class is concerned they focus their needs on the patient. We can't help but get involved with what concerns the nurse. This is true perhaps more so when we're talking about caring for a patient who is dying.

Not uncommonly the students became very upset about the care which their patients were getting.

> One of the students went up to care for a patient. She had been caring for him for a period of time. He had been discharged but readmitted. She did not wear her uniform, was in a lab coat, was in his room. He was comatose. Most people

thought he would die in a very short period of time. She was in the room with him about an hour and a half, and no more nurses came in to take care of him. He needed physical care as well as someone to talk with him. She spent time talking with him, but not giving him physical care because she wasn't in uniform. She was very upset, very concerned about the nurse who was assigned to this patient, who was not coming in. When she approached the nurse about this, initially to help this nurse give this patient care, the nurse would refuse this and cut her off and said she'll be in there in a few minutes. And the few minutes became half an hour, or an hour later. Much of this discussion was related to how the nurse herself felt about not only what was happening to this patient, but also to this nurse herself.

One key function of these class sessions was to give students the chance to talk about experiences which caused them to become upset, and then to take a second look at the problem after the strong feelings had been expressed.

In general, the teachers expected that the students would get involved in considering their own actions as nurses. One teacher expressed her anticipations thus.

I expect her to really attempt to see what is really going on with the patient, to try to understand, to try to support, to try different things, to pose questions about this, to look at what she's thinking, or what *she* wants, *her* feelings, how she's reacting, how she herself is behaving.

Not surprisingly, the teachers had very satisfying experiences when the students performed according to their expectations. The teachers also became frustrated when students resisted this kind of involvement, "Somehow I'd like to get behind these broad, nonspecific kinds of questions. She doesn't really attempt to, and when you attempt to do this, she just throws up her hands, you know." A teacher who returned to school to learn more about interacting with dying patients found herself searching "everywhere" for support when a patient tried to talk openly with her about his forthcoming death.

I had finished taking care of one patient who had been discharged, and then I had been working with another patient for about four or five days, and I had really been making some progress with him. By the time I got to seminar that day I thought, "My God, if somebody doesn't stop long enough for me to talk so that I can tell them about this thing, I'm going to flip." The whole morning after the incident I was aware of the fact that I was trying to corner people to talk to them. I tried to corner the head nurse without much success. I had more success with one of the team leaders, but this didn't last too long. Even the social worker—I had probably the most success with the social worker. She would stand and rest against the table like she'd like to take flight somewhere. I was aware that one staff nurse I actually pinned against the wall, and she tried to sneak away from me. When I went to seminar I was there around ten minutes early with "my knife and fork in my hands" practically—the need to get this off my chest.

She spoke about the value of the seminar in this way.

We had the kind of seminar where you could discuss these kinds of things. You could really discuss the problem, feel helpless, this was the way you felt, and it was acceptable. You live through the problem until you got it resolved. I felt that a lot of this was the teacher's leadership in the class, and part of it was, I suppose it had to do with myself. I took the course because I knew that I had to get more experience in this kind of thing so I felt that I needed to work through problems and get these experiences myself. I really felt I was getting the experiences.

For this teacher, the seminar provided the means whereby she clarified her role in working with dying patients.

Through direct experiences with dying patients, this teacher also became sharply aware of the nurse's need for support when working with these patients.

The thing that struck me most is the amount of support that I felt I needed, and that I could recognize that the staff would also need this kind of thing if we really expected this role to be implemented in the job situation.

As this teacher discovered, interacting openly with dying patients is a tension-producing matter. Nurse teachers, like other nurses, find this part of nursing care difficult to provide. Many teachers want help with the problems they meet in teaching about the care of dying patients. However, schools of nursing have not generally been organized to provide them with support and direction in learning how to cope with this serious nursing (and teaching) problem.

The Faculty as Models

In the hospital the teacher serves as a model for the student in one of two ways: by direct performance of nursing activities or by rehearsal (the provision of information in advance). The teacher can demonstrate the practice of nursing while the student observes her in action, or she can provide the student with some expectations of what is likely to happen in a given situation and what nursing behaviors might appropriately be used. As far as death and dying are concerned, the evidence suggests that the model offered by the faculty is relatively clear-cut for some aspects of nursing practice and quite ambiguous for others. The physical components of care tend to be explicit. The psychological aspects are uncertain.

That many clinical instructors are not themselves comfortable in the presence of death is demonstrated by the commonly used teaching practice of assigning the student to carry out postmortem body care with a staff member rather then assisting the student personally. When the teacher avoids direct contact with the dying situation or appears ill at ease when confronted by it, the student recognizes that the teacher is not comfortable in coping with the assignment. As one student put it, "She was quite nervous and tense. She seemed like she didn't know what to do either, and she explained later that this was the reaction of a lot of people." The model many teachers offer is one emphasizing avoidance of the dying patient, and what the students learn about this part of nursing often comes from other sources.

Sometimes the students see a discrepancy between what the teacher describes as good nursing and what they see her doing in practice. As one student said,

> I had an instructor who idealized nursing, but when she got to the patient I saw her do things that any normal nurse would do. It knocked me for a blow that she wasn't practicing what she was preaching. When I saw her with the patient I was quite shocked, and this really floored me.

Much of the time, however, the students have no opportunity to see their instructors in interaction with dying patients, nor do they often get specific advice on how to talk with these patients and their families. Although the students are offered a general mandate to provide psychological care and support, they infrequently see their teachers providing these kinds of services to patients. A major reason is that the teachers do not really know what to do. As one young teacher said when the student asked her how to talk with dying patients, "Since I am pretty upset myself, I really don't know what to tell them."

What to say, and how to say it, to dying patients and their families is usually not taught by most teachers, but there is another omission which is also important. Perhaps because of the do-it-yourself phenomenon, there is a tendency among nurse teachers to limit the amount of information they give to students about their patients. Rather there is the expectation that the student should pick up what is important on her own. Put differently, the student often begins a patient assignment without any rehearsal as to the expected and unexpected events which might take place. A teacher may assign a terminal patient because he is critically ill, but she is unlikely to talk in advance about the possibility of his dying. Thus the responsibility for defining the dying patient's status is left to the student, who may or may not be able medically, or prepared psychologically, to recognize the situation. Many untoward experiences with dying patients take place because the teachers do not make a practice of forewarning students that death, either expected or unexpected, may occur.

They fail to do so because they themselves do not usually define the assignment in these terms.

That nurse teachers are ill at ease in a situation where death may result is perhaps best illustrated by the behavior of a faculty group when a student in the school was found to have a malignancy, and an uncertain future. The decision was made that she be permitted to complete her schooling, but only one teacher was able to talk directly to the student about her illness. The others avoided direct discussion, at the same time reprimanding the teacher in question for failing to offer special consideration to the student. The majority of the faculty talked as though the student would recover but acted as though they were not sure, by being overly solicitous or by avoiding direct personal contact with her. As nurses often do when faced with a situation which causes them to feel uncomfortable and helpless, these teachers responded by withdrawing from interactions which might activate these feelings. They responded to the diagnosis by enforcing a kind of "protective" social isolationism around the student.[12]

These teachers responded to a situation where death might result in much the same way as do groups of laymen when confronted with a similar predicament. There was a general tendency to treat the student like an invalid who needed special privileges, rather than like an ordinary student. Of course, these teachers were not necessarily functioning as nurses, but they did serve as nurse models for the students to observe.

A Résumé

Teachers in schools of nursing work in an environment in which change is a constant factor. It is an environment characterized by unrest and tension stemming in part from changes in medical technology, changes in relationships between physi-

[12] See Jeanne C. Quint, "Institutionalized Practices of Information Control," *Psychiatry*, 28 (May, 1965), pp. 119–132, for an account of some practices used by doctors and nurses to manage their interaction with cancer patients.

cians and nurses, changes in relationships between educators and practitioners of nursing, and effects of student-centered teaching on what is expected of teachers by schools of nursing. The individual teacher's perspective on teaching about death is a derivative of several factors, especially the clinical setting in which she teaches and her expectations as a nurse and as a teacher. In determining what happens to students when they encounter dying patients on the wards, three different teacher perspectives are very influential—the inexperienced teacher, the unaware teacher, and the concerned teacher.

Helping students while they learn to interact more openly with dying patients is tension-producing and difficult teaching. In general, teachers who do so must find support for themselves on an *ad hoc* basis because schools of nursing have not been organized to provide "backstopping" facilities for the instructional staff. As models of nursing practice, many teachers show themselves to be ill at ease in the presence of death. Notwithstanding the heavy emphasis given to the psychological care of patients, relatively few teachers are themselves able to talk openly and comfortably with dying patients. For the most part, the interaction model the teachers present is one emphasizing avoidance of dying patients. The students, however, can seldom avoid interacting and conversing with the patients to whom they are assigned. The next chapter describes what happens when the students get into conversation with dying patients.

Chapter 4 | Conversations with Dying Patients

Student's encounters with dying patients can sometimes result in serious and upsetting conversations. Patients may know they are dying and wish to talk about it. Patients may suspect they are dying and be testing another's knowledge of it. Patients may be in error and still want to talk about it. They may not know they are dying; but if the student does, she must make certain that she does not say or do anything during conversations to rouse their suspicions. Patients who precipitate conversational dilemmas for students are not necessarily dying in the medically defined sense of "being terminal," although some may be. They are often persons who have a personal interest in death at that time.[1]

[1] More appropriately, this chapter is concerned with conversations between nurse students and persons who are living with a disease carrying fatal connotations or who are threatened by the possibility of sudden death or of a particular way of dying.

Under some conditions talk with dying patients can be relatively easy. Under other circumstances it can be extremely difficult, and typically it is. At best, however, conversations with dying patients are hazardous enterprises because of the unstable nature of these conversations. They typically take place under conditions which can easily change and alter either the context of the interaction or the subject matter under discussion—thus endangering the student's equanimity. Surprise is a frequent component in many critical encounters, and some incidents are meaningful to students precisely because there is no forewarning. In sharp contrast, other incidents exert an influence so subtle that it is not recognized either by the students or by their teachers. These latter incidents play an important part in the socialization process by which students learn how to define patients in general and how to control delicate work situations which threaten to get out of hand.[2] (The students are not always successful in maintaining the control, as will be pointed out later.) Before turning to the specific influence brought about through early encounters with dying patients, it is well to consider first the relative importance of conversation with patients in general, and the rules which govern this aspect of nursing practice.

Rules Governing Professional Conversation

All professional schools provide sets of rules governing practitioner-client relationships, and schools of nursing are no exception. Such rules derive from legal, ethical, and authoritative sources governing "accepted" standards of good practice, as well as relationships with other professionals and the society as a whole. Some rules are explicit and set well-defined limits of responsibility. Thus it is the physician's prerogative and responsibility to tell the patient

[2] As used here, the term *socialization* refers to a process whereby an individual learns to perform in a given role. Renee C. Fox, in *Experiment Perilous* (New York: Free Press, 1959), p. 235, defines the term as follows, "Stated in more formal sociological terms, 'socialization' consists of the processes of learning through which an individual acquires the knowledge, skills, attitudes, values, and behavior patterns which will enable and motivate him to perform a role in a socially acceptable fashion."

his diagnosis and prognosis. By comparison, other rules are generalized and vague; for instance, the directive to provide psychological care is subject to somewhat different interpretations and methods of implementation.

The rules governing conversation with patients are less explicit than the rules governing physical care and technical procedures. There are some exceptions, of course, but generally speaking the management of conversation is left to the commonsense determination of the nurse. Even specific directives—such as the commitment to teach patients—emphasize the content to be taught, but include few well-defined statements on how to proceed or when to start.[3] Some teachers stress the nurse's role in encouraging patients to express their feelings, but offer few explicit guidelines for determining when this action is or is not appropriate for the nurse.[4] Some teachers do offer specific advice about talking with patients, often to facilitate the students' performance of other nursing tasks. One teacher commented about the matter,

> I think that the students do have difficulty learning how to talk to patients as a whole, and how to phrase conversation so that they can be more or less the leader of the situation. This is something that I try to help them develop. When they say to a patient, "Do you want your bath now?" I suggest they try something like, "Well, you've had your breakfast, let's get along with your bath." In some instances the younger students

[3] The critical importance of such factors as the timing of instruction, the assignment of a specific person to do the job, and the basic "facts" which help patients to understand what lies ahead for them has been explicitly detailed for one group of patients. The results of a systematic method of preoperative instruction for patients facing open-heart surgery are described by Filomena Fanelli Varvaro in "Teaching the Patient About Open Heart Surgery," *American Journal of Nursing*, 65 (October, 1965), pp. 111–115.

[4] Bursten and Diers suggest that the literature on patient-centered nursing may have given undue stress to the importance of helping the patient clarify and express his feelings, without concomitant attention to the value of other aspects of the nurse-patient interaction—hereby fostering the danger that communication with patients becomes a new kind of ritual. Ben Bursten and Donna K. Diers, "Pseudo-Patient-Centered Orientation," *Nursing Forum*, Vol. 3, No. 2 (1964), pp. 38–50.

have difficulty in learning to say no to a patient. They want to do everything the patient wants.

Often, however, the directions given by the teacher are vague, with the exception of those rules which clearly specify the doctor's obligations to the patient.

Initially the teacher is perceived as a major resource for information about handling conversations. In the beginning, students are concerned about what to say if the patient asks about his diagnosis or his treatment. The concern about what to say is commonly triggered by an early assignment (sometimes the first) to a patient with cancer. One student reported her first encounter with a cancer patient in this way.

> One of the first statements she made was that the patient next to her had cancer. She looked at me and whispered, as if it were something to be dreaded. Yet she had already gone through this. She also indicated that the person across from her had cancer, and she was a little concerned about that. She talked about her previous hospital experience, and once said that she hadn't seen the doctor in two weeks. There was a note in the nurses' notes that she was anxious about it because she didn't know. I was kind of worried that she would ask about it because I wouldn't know how to answer.

As was common practice when patient assignments were just beginning, the student turned to a teacher for explicit direction.

> Yes, I went to her (the teacher). I concluded that if she (the patient) did ask, I was to try to find out how she had been told. I would just have to say that I didn't know very much. I don't know too much about patients with cancer. If it were me, I think I would be afraid if I didn't know.

Rather than consulting on an individual basis, the students sometimes bring the subject into a class discussion to get answers on the proper ways of talking with such patients. There are four general strategies that the teachers present: (1) Disclosure of the diagnosis (and dying) is the doctor's prerogative, and "you'll have to ask your doctor" is the chief method for handling direct questions about such matters. (2) Because health teaching is an important part of nursing practice, an emphasis can be placed on preparing the patient to leave the hospital. (3) The nurse can also help patients keep their minds off their troubles by encouraging them to talk about their families or their life outside the hospital, or, perhaps, by initiating some form of occupational therapy. (4) Rather than diverting them from their troubles, the nurse can instead provide them with emotional support by encouraging them to express their feelings at a deeper level. The specific ways of implementing emotional support are not always clear to the students, as the following comment suggests, "Once the patient knows his diagnosis, the nurse supposedly is to help the patient talk about this, come to terms with it, and somehow feel the feelings and thoughts. How you do this, I don't know."

Few teachers are experienced in coping with the delicate conversational nuances which prolonged contacts with dying patients may require, nor are they comfortable in such situations. Consequently, they can offer few suggestions for talking to patients who may be frightened by the prospect of dying. The teacher's direction may even deny the possibility of dying, as the following example clearly shows.

A student was assigned to a man with a myocardial infarct during the critical period following its onset. She was aware of the danger of certain physical complications and defined this assignment as a challenging one, with the important nursing tasks being to keep his mind occupied and to plan for his hospital discharge. In discussing her plans with the teacher, the student asked if it were giving the patient false hope to tell him "things will be better, and you can do more for yourself later." At this time the patient's activities were completely restricted by the doctor's order. Even though the teacher was well aware that the patient's prognosis was viewed as highly unfavorable by the physicians in attendance, she answered "no" to the student's question.

Not only are many of the "rules" for talking with dying patients decided by the individual student, but many of the "rules" for deciding when a patient is dying are also decided by her.[5] During the first year in school, assignments to dying patients play an important part in the development both of the "rules" for knowing when a patient is dying and of the strategies for managing conversations when the patient knows (or does not know) that he is dying.[6]

The Assignment Context and Recognition of Dying

When students first begin their patient assignments, they are often concerned about what to say if the patient starts to talk about a subject like dying. A student made these comments about the first day on a ward.

> One girl does have a cancer patient, and it doesn't look too promising right now. The patient's had previous operations on this. Our group, the three of us and the instructor, discussed this when we left the floor. I think all of us were concerned about how to handle the patient's apprehensions and anxieties because evidently the patient doesn't know the real definition of her condition. Not knowing how much she knows, we don't know how much to convey to her that we know.

[5] The development of expectations about dying is considered more fully in Chapter 6. For a more general discussion of the sociological perspective on dying as a definitional problem, readers are referred to Barney G. Glaser and Anselm L. Strauss, *Awareness of Dying* (Chicago: Aldine, 1965), pp. 16–26.

[6] The interaction which occurs between a nurse and a dying patient is guided by the patient's and the nurse's awareness of his dying state. There are four commonly recurring situations (referred to as awareness contexts) observed in the hospital. They are (1) *closed awareness*—the situation in which the patient does not recognize his impending death though everyone else does (or when the patient does, but the nurse may not); (2) *suspected awareness*—the situation in which the patient suspects that he is dying and tries to confirm his suspicions; (3) *mutual pretense awareness*—the situation in which both the patient and the others define him as dying, but each pretends that the other does not know; and (4) *open awareness*—the situation in which both the staff and the patient define him as dying, are aware of the other's definition, and are relatively open in their conversation and actions. See *ibid.*, pp. 9–13.

The students are actually concerned about two problems—recognizing that a patient is dying and being able to cope with conversations about difficult subjects (of which dying is only one).

In the beginning, assignments are usually chosen to protect the students from extremely difficult nursing problems. At the same time, these experiences offer them opportunities to learn conversational strategies through direct practice and through observation of others. During the first year much time is devoted to formal class work and less time is given to clinical practice. What few hours the student does spend with each patient are likely to be focused on technical practice, and faculty supervision is frequent. The custom of assigning students to patients for only one or two days limits the opportunity for serious conversation by restricting the time available for it. However, these brief periods give students the chance to test different conversational approaches and to evaluate their worth.

New students are prone to seek advice on what to do from others whom they see as "knowledgeable": older nursing students, students from related fields (medicine or dentistry), classmates, nurses in practice, and family members, particularly if they are nurses or doctors. Not uncommonly, the students check out in advance the "rules" given in the hospital procedure book or in the standard nursing texts.

> We have a nursing manual, and it has a page on care of a patient after death. I think this was very interesting to all of us about realizing what the responsibilities of a nurse are—preparation of the body, tagging, and escorting to the morgue, proper position, and things you really don't think about in relationship to death in our culture. That's why I see it as a formal kind of ritual you might say. I think this starts right after death in preparation by the nurse to escort the body—it was interesting. You really don't think about it.

Another kind of planning is in the form of speculating about what to say if a patient asks an awkward question. This type of strategy session usually takes place in the residence hall in preparation for the following day.

We were talking about it last night, as to what she could possibly say. We only came up with the fact that we would all have to be patient until the testing results came through, and then we could find a definite course of action. Other than this, there's not much you could really say.

Classmates who have worked in hospitals prior to becoming students are considered particularly knowledgeable authorities, and some find themselves serving as "mother hen" to less experienced colleagues. Once in the hospital, the student can observe the words and actions of others. She can overhear other nurses talking with patients and can profit from their mistakes and successes. She can listen to the teacher talking with another student and can pick up useful cues about what to do and what not to do. No longer does she rely principally on the instructor, for she can now turn directly to the hospital staff for assistance.

The patient assignment has a characteristic which permits students to engage in a wide range of conversational experimentation. A great many conversations between students and patients take place when others are not present. Conversation between any two people is generally quite different from that which occurs when others are in the room—and particularly "others" who represent authority to one or both of the interactants. Because these conversations with patients are often not observed, the student has considerable control over what she does and what she reports; she can decide whether or not to share it and, perhaps equally important, with whom. The one-to-one conversation is important for yet another reason. It is in this context that the student is most likely to encounter conversational difficulties with patients who are dying.

Some important "rules" become apparent during the early weeks on the wards. The students learn that instructors, for the most part, do not hold them accountable for their conversations with patients. When a student approaches a teacher for advice about a conversational problem, she is likely to be told, "You'll have to do it yourself," or, "Every case is individual." She may be referred to a book on interviewing. Occasionally the students can see and hear their teachers interacting with patients, and the reactions are favorable: "It was so easy for her to get the patient to talk." On other occasions, the student is disappointed: "She wasn't any more comfortable or any better than other nurses." There is a progressive shift away from asking instructors for advice and an increased reliance on staff nurses and other students. The students soon recognize the need for getting advance information about patients, and ward personnel who can fulfill this function are readily identified. Sometimes the information is shared through the student grapevine.

The assignment context in which students are introduced to patient assignments often helps prevent the student from recognizing when a patient is dying. Although the student is expected to know the patient's diagnosis, she is left to draw her own conclusions about the likelihood of death. Under these circumstances the student slips easily into the practice of considering patients recoverable. Certain early encounters with patients and staff play an important part in fostering the practice of keeping oneself unaware of the possibility that a patient can be classified as dying. In the beginning, students are prone to ask the doctor directly about a patient's prognosis and can be shocked to learn that nothing more can be done. A student reported these reactions after talking with a physician.

It was just a feeling as though the whole floor had been taken out from under me. He told me that the cancer had gone all the way. I had suspected it, and I had even discussed the case with a medical student who suggested this. But I just ignored it from him. But this confirmed it when the doctor told me. It really hit hard—hit home.

That whole day I was more sensitive to everything that was going on around me. Which is unusual for me. When I was in psychology class, I felt more. I was more sensitive to the emotional picture, and it wasn't until that evening that I snapped out of it.

As all nurses know, it is one thing to read *cancer* on the chart; it is quite another to hear the doctor say *there is nothing more we can do*. Many students discontinue this practice of querying the doctor because it is upsetting to know that no cure is possible, and teachers seldom hold them accountable for knowing it.

The first assignment to a patient with cancer is often an important one. To their surprise, students find that patients with cancer do not necessarily initiate conversation about cancer or dying. Other students find—as did one—that asking a patient what the doctor had told him brought forth a surprise announcement, "Things don't look too good." To avoid this unforeseen situation which is likely to be both upsetting and difficult to manage conversationally, students are likely to make minimal use of the direct question. From these assignments students can also learn strategies for coping with unexpected remarks. Quite rapidly they find that silence can be a particularly effective way of deflecting the unwanted question or comment. Sometimes an innocuous comment can successfully parry a penetrating question. In one situation a man with a grotesque skin cancer tested a young student by asking her how his wound looked. She found that the comment, "It doesn't look bad. I would rather look at that than a skinned knee," averted further discussion of the topic.

Not all encounters provide such simple answers. Sometimes students decide *what not to do* as an aftermath of an incident, as the following episode shows. A student was assigned to a cancer patient shortly after the doctor had informed the woman of her poor prognosis. The student encouraged the patient to talk and on the second day of the assignment found herself quite unprepared to handle the situation when the woman began to cry. As a consequence, this student decided that it was better to let patients take the initiative in deciding what to discuss.

Students also find that patients who are defined as dying do not always "look dying," nor do they necessarily act as though they are about to have their lives brought to an end.

> We had a fourteen-year-old boy with a terminal diagnosis. He came in for a biopsy of a tumor of the leg, which was cancer and had metastasized. They were originally going to do radical surgery but decided that it would be foolish to do because the boy had not long to live. This was very difficult because he

was extremely healthy looking, and a healthy acting person. He enjoyed talking about sports. He wanted to fix up the student nurses with his uncle for a date. He was marvelous with the other children, and he didn't seem ill at all.

Out of experiences such as these, some students become aware of the protective value of knowing in advance that a patient is categorized as dying.

It is not only patients with cancer who provide these kinds of experiences, but they provide a great many. From these and similar incidents students construct a picture of how patients generally behave in hospitals and what kinds of surprise conversations can be met. Concomitantly, they find that certain techniques are effective for avoiding conversational difficulties or for cutting them short. Social conversation is a useful technique for eluding talk about distressing topics and is generally successful unless the patient is terribly upset and forces the issue. Such an unexpected encounter can happen to anyone at any time, but students learn early to guard against the possibility in several ways—getting advance warning about patients, avoiding extra time with a potentially dangerous talker, bringing someone else into the room, directing the patient's attention to the procedures to be undergone. As young adults they are already familiar with many ways of controlling awkward conversation, and they can easily put these into practice. Also, the assignment context permits the student to make many choices which control the amount of time spent with patients.

Obviously the students cannot completely protect themselves from awkward or difficult conversations with dying patients, but they have many conversations which are not in the least troublesome. Sometimes the nondifficult conversation occurs when the student knows that a patient is dying. Often, however, the student is quite unaware that the patient falls into this classification. As will become clear later, the degree of vulnerability to conversations which pose problems for the student is less a function of awareness of dying *per se* than of the *timing* of becoming aware and the *mode* by which knowledge about dying is conveyed.

Awareness and Nondifficult Conversation

The Student Does Not Know

Students do not encounter conversational difficulties with some patients simply because the students do not know that the patients are dying, and nothing happens to change their awareness of the situation. Sometimes the patients themselves do not know they are dying. In some instances when they have been told, they do not care to talk about it. Frequently students move out of the picture quite unaware of the death potential. The hopeful atmosphere common in hospitals serves not only to play down the importance of dying but also to keep its presence hidden, especially from newcomers. The conversation may represent no special problem to the student—though the extent to which some patients talk about their personal problems often comes as a surprise.

> Then she began to tell me about her marital problems. She told me that she hadn't been able to get pregnant and had gone to the doctor. She tried to get her husband to go to the doctor, but he wouldn't—"Just a big, dumb Swede." I was surprised when she talked to me about this. I didn't expect it.

Many conversations, however, are quite social in nature and easily forgotten.

The inexperienced student may not suspect dying because her limited knowledge prevents her from recognizing the possibility. On the other hand, the advanced student may not suspect because she is already in the habit of treating all patients as recoverable. In either case the student is likely to remain unaware of the dying status when the patient assignment is of short duration and her attention is directed to other matters. Students are assigned to many patients whose diagnoses and prognoses carry "death anticipations," but these patients are usually not defined as dying by the nursing staff or by teachers. Persons facing major surgery or extensive diagnostic testing, for example, are often concerned about what the doctor will find and what the future holds for them.

Sometimes the student may not know the patient is dying, but the patient does and makes efforts to talk about it. The student may not recognize the patient's words either as a clue that death is a possibility or as an invitation to talk about the matter. A specific example will illustrate the point. A first-year student was assigned to a patient facing cardiac surgery on the following day. The student was primarily concerned with teaching the patient how to breathe during the postoperative period, when deep breathing would be a difficult and painful process. During the discussion the patient commented, "I know that God meant this operation to be, that he wanted me to live through it." The student did not know what to say in response and returned to her teaching. The student did not recognize this statement as an indication that the woman might want to talk about the possibility of dying.[7] Furthermore, the patient's statement did not increase the student's awareness that this woman conceivably could die during the surgery. Her death on the operating room table came as a complete surprise. The student learned of the death only when she called the intensive-care unit several days later to inquire about the patient's welfare. The student was not expecting such an outcome, and described her reaction in this way.

> I think it was probably because I hadn't had any contact before with someone dying on the operating table. A lot of times these things happen, you know. I think that death is something that you sort of figure, it's there but you don't exactly figure that it would happen to your best friend or to a patient you have taken care of. She seemed so well and walking around. I think I would have had a different attitude if it had been a patient, like one on a medical floor, or someone who I had taken care of who was slowly slipping. But the idea that she was perfectly well when I left the floor, and I wasn't

[7] What this comment actually meant to the patient can only be conjectured.

back for three or four days before I checked it. When I finally found out that she had died, it didn't register particularly. It's unreal. And I had assumed that she would be in ICU anyway, so there would be no reason why I would have found her on the ward.

This kind of situation—failure to recognize the possibility of dying—is likely to happen under several circumstances. The student is new and lacking in experience. The patient looks healthy. Neither teacher nor staff warn the student of the possibility of death. The student's attention is directed to other matters. The assignment is extremely brief. In the preceding instance, the student learned of the patient's dying status as a postassignment phenomenon. Many students engage in conversation with dying patients under similar circumstances but never realize that the patients are trying to talk about their fears of dying. The assignments change and the students move on uninformed of the patients' desires (or dying status). The context of awareness remains "closed" (with the students as the innocent parties).

The Student Knows

Sometimes the student knows the patient is dying, but the patient does not know (also a closed awareness context). This situation can occur when patients with such potentially fatal diseases as cancer have not been told the diagnosis and are not yet sick enough to ask questions which might be difficult to answer. Patients themselves can make talk easy by chatting about social matters or by expressing interest in the nurse's affairs. Students in this context not uncommonly guide the conversation away from talk about the illness, or they limit the time spent with the patient.

As long as the patient does not suspect or is content to let things be as they are, conversation can be relatively easy. The more clues the patient has to arouse his suspicions, the more unstable the the situation is conversationally, and the more the student must guard her words (suspected awareness context). This situation may be easy to maintain for short periods of time, but it can be extremely difficult when an assignment is extended and other conditions change concurrently.

Sometimes both the student and the patient know that he is dying, but they engage in mutual pretense and talk about other matters.[8] This type of exchange is likely to occur when the student and patient are new to one another, when the patient has come to terms with his impending death, and when the patient is not distressed by pain or upset by other matters. In such an interaction, neither participant makes an effort to find out directly what the other knows, although both may suspect; nor does either openly acknowledge his own state of awareness. One student described an assignment in the following words.

> This was just sort of conveyed between us. I didn't come right out and say, and she just sort of knew. The next four or five days she had progressively gotten worse. She was in bed most of the time, and was vomiting a good deal. The nurse had told me that she probably wouldn't have long to live, even though the doctor had said that she had six months. There wasn't much verbal communication from that point on, because she was extremely tired and weak. Due to all this vomiting, she didn't have much time to sleep. She told me one time that it was more comforting to her to have someone just there, rather than to have someone to talk to her. So I just stayed there as much as I could, and maybe put my hand on her shoulder just to let her know that I was with her.

Because the circumstances underlying the situation can change rapidly, and frequently do, the game of mutual pretense has limited chances of continuing when assignments are prolonged. For one thing, it simply becomes extremely awkward for two people to behave as though everything were fine when both know otherwise and see each other day after day. Again, both patient and student may know that the patient is dying, but the patient may not be

[8] See Glaser and Strauss, *op. cit.*, pp. 64–78, for a general discussion of this kind of interaction.

sure the student knows and does not discuss it with her. Alternately, he may simply act out of compassion for the student who is "so young."

In the situations described thus far, the conversations were relatively easy because they did not focus directly on dying or its possibility. Even open talk related to death is not necessarily difficult if the topics raised by the patient are not troublesome for the student. A student told the following story about an assignment.

> Afterwards I had a great sense of achievement with her. She was a young woman of about forty-four, and she had a young daughter of ten. I had her for two days (two mornings), and the first day I kind of, you know, felt my way along in the situation. My instructor had me do what we call a process recording. That night I went over it with my instructor, and we looked at the patient's needs and all, so I had a pretty good idea of the patient's emotional needs and questions and recurrent scenes and all.

> The second day she talked quite frequently about after her death—who would iron her husband's shirts and how her daughter would go to college. She wanted her daughter to be sure to go to college. I was able to give her suggestions about the college facilities that apparently she was not aware of. I felt a sense of accomplishment here.

Open talk about death is not difficult if the patient is relaxed about the matter, and the topic is a peripheral one—in this instance, a mother's concerns for her child's future. Also, the same student was able to perform a concrete act of assistance, a factor which reduced the sense of hopelessness so commonly felt by students when they talk with dying patients.

Protection Through Short and Multiple Assignments

The preceding assignment might have changed in character and in emotional tone had it continued beyond two days. Once more, the significance of the short assignment as a prime condition for "easy" conversation becomes apparent, though other conditions may vary.

When students are assigned to many patients, the short assignment offers few conversational risks. The student has less time to devote to each patient, therefore less time for talk, and she has access to many strategies for removing herself from potentially difficult situations. Student interest is frequently focused on learning nursing techniques and on completing assignments within a prescribed time period, and instructor supervision is likely to be spread thin to accommodate the needs of other students. Not uncommonly there is less emphasis given to the significance of nurse-patient conversation in this assignment context, and students are not pushed to experiment with it. Obviously, troubled patients can initiate "death" conversation under these circumstances, but students have many avenues available for avoiding situations they cannot handle. They have other patients to serve, other tasks to finish, and classes to attend. As a last resort a student can always ask for an assignment change. Under the multiple-patient assignment, which is like the staff nurse work assignment, students less frequently get into conversational dilemmas of their own making.

Awareness and Difficult Conversations

Each situation previously described carries the potential for difficult conversation if one or more conditions change. Thus the patient may learn the truth and announce his dying status to the unsuspecting student. The surprise announcement is difficult at best, but can be worse if the patient's behavior is also disturbing. The following incident illustrates this point.

A young student was giving morning care to a man who quite suddenly blurted out that he was dying, that there was nothing more she could do. He brusquely told her to leave the room. Taken aback, the student went to her teacher, who told her to do whatever she thought best. Returning to the patient, the student tried to explain that the treatment was necessary. He responded,

"Don't fool me; I don't want it." The student completed the treatment, but the assignment was a "terrible experience" because he never stopped telling her to get out of his sight.

The patient who does not know may become suspicious when he notes certain physical changes in himself and may ask the student probing questions that she finds difficult to parry. The doctor may tell the patient he is dying, yet the student may not know this has occurred and may continue to block the patient's conversational overtures. The patient who knows he is dying may change his behavior pattern, as can happen when pain becomes worse or family pressures impinge on him so heavily that he must blow off to someone. He may no longer pretend that he is getting well, but begin to talk about death in general, or his own in particular. The patient who has talked serenely about leaving his family behind may suddenly start talking about his fear of dying or his concern about pain and what the end will be like. He may become very agitated and openly talk about suicide. Whether influenced by a change in awareness of his dying status or by changes in other circumstances which affect his living, the dying patient may need to talk about matters that are important to him. These topics, however, can be very upsetting to the student.

Some difficult conversations take place because students initiate talk which gets out of hand. The student herself may unknowingly precipitate a crisis by asking the wrong question or by making what she thought was an innocent comment. In the middle of an assignment the student may learn that the patient is dying and then find herself speechless in a situation which formerly posed no problems. Students who encourage dying patients to verbalize or to express their feelings can find themselves very upset by the unforeseen consequences of using this approach. Thus even a short assignment can be conversationally hazardous for any student who encourages patients to talk about their real concerns.

Sometimes an assignment is difficult not because of the conversation but because the patient will not talk at all. Similarly, a student may find it difficult to carry on when a patient is openly hostile, highly critical of her actions, or constantly complaining. A student reported these reactions to her first patient assignment.

> I was shaking so much by this time that I was having a little trouble with the thermometer, so the instructor stayed with me. When I inserted it and told him I would have to hold it in place for five minutes, she left. Well, I was too concerned with myself to attempt any conversation with the patient, particularly after such a rebuff that I had gotten. He just turned his face away and made no conversation whatsoever. It wasn't until about a week later, in a conference in which we were discussing how one determines levels of illness and wellness, that I found out this man was a terminal patient about to die. At this time I felt guilty for thinking he was such a terrible old man, nasty and so on.

This type of interaction is difficult for any young student, and particularly one who is unsure of herself. It can be a traumatic event when it takes place as part of the first patient assignment.

As can easily be seen, the conversation becomes hazardous whenever a patient attempts to shift from one awareness context to another, whether this be from closed to open or suspected, from mutual pretense to open, or from suspected to open. In addition, an open awareness context without danger can unexpectedly become a perilous enterprise. The student can also cause a change in awareness context, sometimes purposefully and sometimes inadvertently, thereby suddenly finding herself faced with a situation that has gone completely out of control.

The shifts in awareness context occur with greater frequency when prolonged assignments are used. Even when the multiple assignment (usually low in risk) is employed, the conversational hazards increase when the assignment time is extended for several weeks. A student is less able to define a dying patient as nondying through such a lengthy period, and she is not well protected from personal involvement with the patient and his family. Prolonged contact increases the possibility that a patient may initiate efforts to talk openly about his dying. Maintaining the pretense that the patient will recover becomes increasing difficult for both him and the student as physical signs indicate otherwise.

Conversations Described as Difficult

It is now easy to understand why there are two general classes of conversations students find very difficult. First, there are the conversations to be handled when the student is assigned to a dying patient who is not to be told the truth about his condition, yet he suspects the truth. Then there are the hazards when patients want to talk openly about their own deaths, and the students cannot tolerate either the topic being discussed or the patient's behavior, or both together.

Conversations and the Nondisclosure Assignment

When the student is assigned to a patient who is not to be told his diagnosis, she is faced with several distressing problems. She must converse with the patient without giving him any clues which might reveal his true condition. This task becomes extremely difficult, if not almost impossible, when the patient suspects and asks direct questions. One student described the problem in this way.

> When I would walk into her room, she would say, "I wonder why I have pain in this region or that region." If I knew that she was aware of what her diagnosis was, I would be able to explain a little bit, but she didn't. I was almost afraid to say anything because I didn't know if I would slip.

The much-used phrase *you'll have to ask your doctor* may not stop the patient's efforts to get information from the student. Frequently the student is primary recipient of a patient's concerns because the hospital nurses tend to withdraw from patients who press them for the "facts." Conversational pretense becomes particularly awkward when the patient's physical condition is obviously deteriorating, or when relatives gather in the room as though preparing for a wake. A student commented about an assignment which was a "great strain."

She kept referring to all those purple bruises, and every time you'd walk in she'd say, "Why do I have these bruises?" She had two conditions (I can't remember what the other one was) but it certainly wasn't something that would cause these bruises. It just didn't correlate to the point where, if it were you or I, we would suspect something was seriously wrong. She was always asking questions. You always had to be on your guard.

In addition, the student may have trouble with her own feelings if she thinks patients have the right to know what is happening to them, as the following incident suggests.

Some of my friends are taking care of this man since I left. His wife refused to let him know he is dying, and I think it is pretty wrong. She has him so subjugated and she has done so many things. I think he might want to do things a little differently if he knew he was dying.

Like the ward nurses, the student often finds herself caught between the patient and his doctor and family. Sometimes the patient, informed by signs and symptoms, may well suspect a certain diagnosis and will ask pertinent questions which must be answered by not saying anything which would disclose his condition. As one student observed, "Here you have a fight between the doctor who doesn't want you to tell her and the patient who wants to know. Where do you talk first?" The student who does give information to a patient, either accidentally or purposefully, may have the added problem of facing an angry physician.

Nondisclosure problems can be even worse if the patient is emotionally disturbed, as the following episode illustrates. A first-year student was assigned to a woman who had gone to surgery on the previous day for a breast biopsy. The patient had previously had one breast removed for cancer and was suspicious of what the doctors had found. The student knew that the biopsy was positive for cancer, but she also knew that the surgeon had not yet talked to the patient. This student had been told by a teacher that she could not use the word *cancer* until the doctor himself had used it with the patient. One of her classmates described what took place.

Anyway Mary attempted to talk to this woman about it, but the woman was incapable of it. She just kept saying, "I want to die, I want to die, but I cannot ask you to do this. I can't ask you to let me die because you are a student, and you can't do it." Then she began to cry and Mary was completely dismayed. You know, what will I do now? Well, she had to leave the room and go and cry herself. Then she returned and asked the woman if she wanted to talk about it. The woman said "no" and started to cry again. Mary said, "I will stay with you, if you would like," and the woman said, "yes." So she just stayed with her and held her hand.

The student herself found the assignment a very upsetting experience, and she did not know how to cope with it. Part of her difficulty stemmed directly from the paradoxical assignment with its two conflicting directives. (See Chapter 3, pp. 65–66.)

Tension-Producing Topics of Conversation

The preceding incident clearly demonstrates the two conditions which make open talk about death a difficult problem—the upset patient and tension-producing subject matter. When patients aware of their coming deaths talk about peripheral topics, such as reminiscing about the past, students have little difficulty either in listening or in engaging in repartee. However, the student and many others find themselves at a loss for words when the patient focuses directly on the central issue of his personal death—for instance, when he says, "I want to get it over with now." The student is faced with handling her own reactions (feelings of helplessness and hopelessness, or a sense of frustration) when a patient openly expresses the wish to die. As one student commented, "When she talked about death, I always got anxious."

Another particularly distressing assignment is one in which the patient talks openly about his death on one day, yet makes plans to leave the hospital on the next. In this situation it may not be talk about death which poses problems, but rather deciding what to say in response to the erroneously hopeful plans for recovery.

When the patient swings from hopeful talk on one occasion to deep despair the next, the problem of maintaining conversational equilibrium is a strain. The student may well feel inadequate and uncomfortable. She is likely to remember the assignment as an unhappy and emotionally draining experience.

The topics which give students the greatest difficulty are those that are likely to be extremely important to the dying patient— the time of his death, the manner of his dying, and the desire to bring closure to his life. The patient may wonder when he will die, and whether he will be conscious until the end. He may worry that the pain will get worse, with no relief available to him. He may want to die quietly without the use of extensive life-prolonging measures as the end draws near. He may want to talk openly about dying so that he can say good-bye to his family and the staff, or to make plans for what will happen after he is gone. A student reported this conversation with a patient.

> She was talking to me in this general area, and finally we got around to the fact that people shouldn't be afraid. I said, "Well, are you afraid?" She said, "Well, I'm afraid but not of death." I said, "Well, what are you afraid of then?" She said, "of the pain," because she felt so much pain now and she was sure as she got worse, she would have a lot more pain. She said the actual dying didn't bother her.

The patient may ask for help in making critical decisions, and the student can view this request as an inappropriate one. A terminal cancer patient was faced with the alternative of going home to die or of taking an experimental drug with no guarantee of cure. In talking with the student assigned to her, the woman kept repeating, "What shall I do? What shall I do?" The student thought that the patient was asking her to make the decision. The student reported her own reactions thus.

> When she said, "I want to die," I kept thinking, "Well, I don't want to die—you couldn't want to die." I was always thinking that she can't mean that, and tighten up. A lot of her comments were what-should-I-do types of things and asking

my advice on what choice she should make, which made me anxious because here was somebody who was older than my mother, who was very intelligent, and who I would normally think of myself as looking up to, she was asking me for help.

To the student this assignment was an exhausting experience.

In some ways, I guess it was a drain on me because I got to like her so much, maybe more than I should have, and I just felt too much I *wish* there were some way I could help her, but I didn't know how. She wanted some answers, and I couldn't give them to her.

Being this close to another person's experience of dying can indeed be an emotionally depleting experience. The tension can be heightened even more if the patient talks about killing himself or makes a direct request to "put me out of my misery."

It should now be abundantly clear that difficult conversations with dying patients have degrees of difficulty depending not so much upon awareness of dying *per se* as upon other features— the timing of the awareness announcement, the conversational constraints imposed by others (the doctor, the family, the teacher), the subject matter pursued, the emotional states of the interactants, the prior experiences of both, and the length of time they are in contact. As was noted earlier in the chapter, prolonged contact between the student and the patient is a critical precursor for conversational problems. There are several other conditions which also lead in this direction.

Conditions Further Maximizing Difficulties

Prolonged Contact

Prolonged contact does not only occur through lengthy patient assignments, but also takes place when students continue to visit their patients after the official assignment has terminated (a practice which is noticeably less common among senior students than among their less-experienced colleagues). Some patients are also in and out of the hospital several times before their final stay, and students can become well acquainted with them under these circumstances. These points are important because the longer a student knows a dying patient, the more likely she is to learn of characteristics that are not observable on brief contact. In the United States such values as youth, beauty, or talent are highly esteemed, and dying patients who embody these characteristics tend to produce feelings of loss in those who are around them. Like others, the student can become vulnerable to feelings of sadness associated with a person's loss to society or to his family, and thereby can increase her susceptibility to involvement in his dying.

Social Loss Reactions

In any society people are esteemed on the basis of personal and social characteristics which carry high value. In this country age is an important condition for assigning high social value. The death of a child or young adult is generally perceived as a greater loss to society than that of an older person who has lived a full life. Each individual has many kinds of characteristics; social class, ethnic group, sex, education, occupation, family background, accomplishment are some that are important. As is true with nurses in general, students respond to patients in terms of the values ascribed to their social characteristics.[9] A person who is young, talented, and personable tends to be more highly valued than one who is old, useless, and disgruntled. When the patient is dying, these characteristics determine the extent to which his death is perceived as a loss (to society or to the family), thus producing feelings of sadness and regret.

A cluster of high social-loss factors usually carries more impact than a single factor, but even one characteristic can assume singular importance if it is personally meaningful to the student. Patients

[9] A more complete discussion of these points is given by Barney G. Glaser and Anselm L. Strauss in "The Social Loss of Dying Patients," *American Journal of Nursing*, **64** (June, 1964), pp. 119–121.

with these highly valued characteristics are potentially risky assignments because student reactions to them can intensify the tragic feelings of *this person's death*. A student reported these reactions, "There was a boy not too long ago—he died of leukemia. His family was completely upset and cried a lot. I found the best thing to do is to cry along with them." By comparison, the same social characteristics can be relatively unimportant factors *if* the student is unaware that the patient is dying.

Sometimes a combination of traits can produce a social-loss "story" which is sad and disturbing. One student described a three-week assignment to a young mother dying of leukemia. The woman's last baby was also in the hospital, where he had been placed when the mother's disease had exacerbated. Much of the patient's conversation centered around her family and stories of the new baby, as relayed by the patient's mother who visited the nursery daily. The patient did not openly talk to the student about dying, but on one occasion burst into tears. The student could only respond with the words, "Is there anything I can do to help?" She described the assignment as "terribly hard" because "there isn't anything I can say or do." She was reacting to a tragic death: a young mother leaving behind small children and a loving husband.

This incident is important for another reason. It illustrates the compounding of involvement which takes place when a student responds, not solely to social loss, but also to factors which are personally significant. In this instance the student was married and had children of her own. She had first become interested in the patient while assigned to give care to her baby. In the student's words, "I think I am closely associated with her. She has a young family."

Certain situations carry a special poignancy, and one of these is talking with children who are dying. In many instances, the youngsters have not been told what is happening and may even be given false information. While visiting each day, the mother of a boy with cancer metastases in the lungs would say, "When your pneumonia gets better, you can come home." Later the boy asked the nurse student, "Why don't I get better?" The student could say nothing, but she wept when she got home.

Personal-Loss Reactions

Personal loss by itself can be troublesome, as when the student identifies with someone her own age. It can be magnified tremendously when the patient is someone she knows. For instance, she unexpectedly finds herself assigned to the boy next door, for whom "nothing more can be done." An entire class can feel the impact of tragedy when one of its members falls victim to an incurable disease.

Inexperienced students in particular are prone to respond to personal and social-loss characteristics by continuing to visit their patients. A student assigned to a fourteen-year-old boy with a malignant leg tumor kept returning to the ward. As another student commented, "She is never able to do what she wants to do, and I don't think she knows what she wants to do, but she is drawn back." Extended contact through such visits does not necessarily lead to disastrous outcomes, and the student may well come through such an experience with a sense of reward for having been able to give support to the patient or to his family. However, these visiting habits can lead to upsetting consequences if the patient dies unexpectedly and, even more so, if the student was involved in serious conversations with him.

For example, a young man facing heart surgery became very dependent on a student who permitted him to talk about how frightened he was. He wanted her to be with him following surgery, but because of other commitments the student was unable to grant his request. When he died several days following the operation, she felt that she had betrayed his trust by not being present during the postoperative period. Students are frequently unaware of the potential hazards in their encounters with patients, and they cannot predict the impact such experiences will have on their feelings. It is the patient's personal and social characteristics which attract the student and are likely to pull her into a close involvement. It is the conversational dilemma, sometimes left unfinished by sudden death, which can perplex and trouble her.

Accountability for Conversations with Dying Patients

An assignment which frequently leads to conversational difficulties is one in which the student has only one patient—known to be dying—with the commitment to focus conversation on the patient's concerns. Graduate students who are assigned to terminal patients for the duration of their hospital stay (often a matter of weeks) invariably encounter problems either in handling the conversation or in coping with their own feelings, but usually both. Basic students can have similar experiences with short assignments if they happen to be assigned during a period when the patient is undergoing an emotional upheaval. It is the commitment to talk with the patient which makes this assignment a particularly dangerous enterprise. When the teacher holds the student accountable for what goes on between her and the patient, the student cannot easily avoid spending time with the patient. (There are, of course, those students whose facile imaginations can manufacture conversations which please the teacher and save the student from painful first-hand experience; but few students are so blessed.) During this assignment the student tends to get into conversational territory which is new for her, and she often makes matters worse by an inappropriate response.

A specific illustration can clarify the latter point. A student was taken by surprise when a patient said, "I think it would be so much better if the doctors would give me a shot and put me to sleep now." Quite unprepared for this comment, the student responded by saying, "But why should they do that. Look at the way you've been joking." The student felt "horrible" when the patient patted her on the hand and said, somewhat sarcastically, "Oh, you're developing a good bedside manner. You'll make a good nurse." The student said of this assignment, "Emotionally it was the hardest week I've ever had with a patient."

The Management of Conversations with Dying Patients

General Tactics

It should now be easy to see that the students must develop tactics for coping with several distinct problems. They need strategies for knowing when patients are dying so that they can be prepared for a variety of eventualities—patients who know they are dying, those who suspect they are dying, and those who do not know they are dying. Stated differently, the students learn ways of discriminating between potentially "safe" and "unsafe" contexts in which they are expected to talk with patients. With experience the students become aware of important resources for getting advance information—the seriously ill list which contains the names of "unsafe" patients; the patient's chart (not always a reliable source, as students rapidly learn); the reports between nurses at change-of-shift time; and staff members who are usually knowledgeable about such matters.

Another problem is that of learning how to prevent safe assignments from becoming unsafe. This means knowing what to do when an awareness context starts to change—for example, indications appear that a closed awareness context is becoming a suspected awareness context. The student needs two kinds of strategies for controlling this type of interaction problem, contact management (ways of minimizing the time spent with the patient) and expression management (ways of managing conversation which threatens to get out of hand). As far as managing contact time, the student can spend little time with the patient, leave the room when the conversation becomes threatening, or have a third party present if at all possible. The conversation itself can be managed by effective use of both verbal and nonverbal interaction techniques—the nonspecific comment, a change of subject, a selective use of the direct question, referral of questions to an authority (the doctor, staff nurses), the plea of ignorance (readily available to the student and the new employee), the use of social conversation, the depersonalization of the patient by not talking to him, or the professional manner which "puts the patient in his place."

Finally, there are guarding tactics that are necessary for dealing with the assignment which is definitely an unsafe enterprise. The same strategies previously listed can be readily used for avoiding some conversational problems. In addition, the student must be wary of other dangers. Among the additional hazards to be avoided are involvement with a patient whose death would be terribly saddening and conversation which provokes feelings of helplessness, hopelessness, or anger. The effect of prior experience on the development of protective strategies clearly shows up when one contrasts the management of patients by experienced and inexperienced students when they are assigned to a ward with many high-risk patients.

The Experienced Student

Experienced students, when confronted with high social-loss patients, behave so as to minimize the possibilities of personal involvement. On one pediatric ward, which housed a high proportion of children with fatal illnesses, these students successfully kept themselves detached by using the following methods. The assignment was defined as nonterminal. Little conversation was initiated with parents about the child's illness. Personal contact with the child and his parents was limited, and extra assignment time with the patients was avoided. Conversation was focused on everyday matters. Instructor help was seldom sought. Even with children who showed obvious signs of physical deterioration, the students were able to keep themselves uninvolved with the children personally by focusing their attention on the disease or treatment process. The students were aided in the process because assignments were short and instructor supervision was scanty.

Although these students were told that support for families with dying children was an important nursing function, they had little direct help from their teacher, and many chose to minimize their contacts with family members. Such behavior was commonly justified by the rationale that it was not fair to families to start something and then not to be present at critical moments. The practice of minimizing contact with families was also used by the hospital staff, e.g., they frequently held staff conferences during visiting hours. Thus these students were supported in their choices by the nurse models they saw in action.

The Inexperienced Student

The inexperienced student in this setting was likely to get herself into trouble because she did not recognize the warning signs of potential involvement, nor was she adept at ignoring them. A specific incident will illustrate the point. A student was assigned for two days to a twelve-year-old boy with lymphosarcoma. She became so involved that she continued to see the boy and his parents in follow-up clinic. There were a number of factors which led to the involvement. During the assignment the student encountered several conditions she was unable to ignore. The patient's swollen neck was an observable sign, and she chose to define him as "terminal." Twice the boy raised questions about why he was admitted to the hospital. The mother was extremely upset and spoke to the student about her fears that his classmates might "tell him something" when he returned to school. The student responded with sadness to the tragedy of a child facing death.

Caught up in these concerns, the student discussed her goals with a teacher who encouraged her to continue working with the family. The student's primary concern was that no one had given the boy a realistic appraisal of what was happening to him. She wanted to protect him from the chance of hearing the bad news from his classmates. The patient was discharged before the student had "accomplished everything," and she felt compelled to see the family again.

While the youngster was hospitalized, the student had several awkward moments during her conversations with him. She wanted very much to ask him questions directly but was afraid he might put her on the spot. In her words, "It is not my place to tell him." In the clinic she found he was "different than in the hospital" and not receptive to talk. However, she did not spend much time with the boy at this time but chose to talk with his mother, because she wanted the mother to tell the boy that he had a serious blood disease. She never knew whether her effort achieved success because other commitments and new interests assumed priority, and she did not maintain her contact with the family.

Compensating for Helpless Feelings

There are several ways by which students counterbalance their feelings of helplessness and inadequacy when talking with dying patients. Although the counterbalancing does not help them manage actual conversation with patients, it does help them get through unavoidable interaction with patients. Some students learn that referral to the chaplain may give some patients the opportunity to talk about their concerns and to come to terms with their impending deaths. The students find, however, that not all patients find comfort in talking to ministers and that some clergymen have difficulty in providing this kind of help to dying patients. Sometimes a social worker is available for referral when a patient indicates he wants to talk more openly about his coming death, and the student makes use of this service. The student can compensate for her personal inadequacies by bringing another human resource to the patient.

Conversation with family members is another technique which seems to assume a special importance when the dying patient is a child, perhaps to atone for the impact of social-loss feelings. The value of this device is that helping the family provides a sense of helpfulness to the nurse student where hopelessness prevailed before.[10] In the example previously described the student tried to help a twelve-year-old boy by encouraging his mother to give him some definite information. These conversations were not easy, and the experience was described as emotionally depleting. At the same time the student had a sense of accomplishment, and she stated, "I helped the parents more this time than I did in the

[10] This statement does not mean that students do not encounter problems in dealing with the families of dying patients, as will become clear in the next chapter.

hospital. Not that I could give them any solutions; this is impossible. But they could express some of their feelings, and I could show them that I cared." Such a strategy can indeed help a family through this period of strain, but the outcome for the patient may be to isolate him further from involvement in and discussions about his own death.

Sometimes a student is well aware that she has helped a dying patient by bringing him into contact with the "right person." For example, she tells the doctor that the patient seems to be asking for more information, and the patient appears more relaxed with himself after he has talked with his physician. However, sometimes the student is unaware that she has provided assistance, as will be indicated in Chapter 7.

Some Conversational Consequences for Students

The Search for Support

When students encounter conversational difficulties, they often turn to persons other than their teachers for counsel. Even those instructors whom students recognize as good listeners usually have little concrete advice to offer. Some may even withdraw from listening because they cannot tolerate talk about death and the strong feelings which tend to be engendered in them by the student's reactions. When students turn to hospital staff for advice about handling certain patients, they are likely to get one of two responses—agreement with the decision the student has already made, or "You seem to be doing fine by yourself." A few students seek out the clergy for support, but eventually most students turn to classmates or boyfriends, using them as sounding boards. Thus, the advice they get and the decisions they make are based primarily on commonsense determinations, combined with trial-and-error experience. Some students pick up tactics vicariously by listening to student colleagues describe their successes and failures, and many finish the first year quite adept at avoiding distressing conversations with patients. Students without an early exposure to the interactional problems associated with dying develop few cues for judging potentially dangerous situations. They are, therefore, prime candidates for encountering conversational difficulties when they are assigned to seriously ill patients at a later time. They are also ill prepared for the emotional impact these experiences usually bring.

The Aftermath of Conversations with Dying Patients

As has been indicated, students can have very positive experiences in talking with dying patients, and also some very difficult ones. The former are frequently remembered with exhilaration, as moments of great success in providing help or comfort. The latter can run the gamut, from being recalled as mildly upsetting or surprising to being remembered as very traumatic, leaving the student with doubts about herself and uncertainties about what to do in the future.

It is not uncommon for nurse students to attach a cause-and-effect relationship between their conversations with dying patients and the events which take place following them. Some may even blame themselves for the patient's death. In one instance, for example, a patient with inoperable cancer pushed very hard to learn the truth about her condition from the student. The latter took this request to the physician, who then told the patient about her incurable condition. When the patient suddenly developed complications and died within three days, the student blamed herself for having instigated the announcement. Another student can blame herself if a patient who knows he is dying indicates a readiness to talk, yet he dies before the student is psychologically ready to talk with him.

These conversational experiences are upsetting at the time, but they can also serve as important turning points if the students have someone available to help them live through these difficult periods—and particularly when the listeners clarify the positive as well as the less positive consequences of interactions with patients. The few nurse students who learned to talk more openly and comfortably with dying patients had someone to whom they consistently turned for support and guidance when they encountered these difficult problems. As a result, and with the passage of time, they were able to view their actions within a more realistic and less self-critical framework.

There is another reaction which the students do not anticipate, the intensity of their feelings of grief when they become involved with a dying patient. Not only are these reactions personally disturbing, but also they often cause the student to experience conflict within herself because the social role of bereaved person is incongruent with the social role of nurse, as defined by the norms of hospital culture.[11] Just as students were helped by talking about difficult conversations, so also were they helped when they could openly express the many and varied feelings which accompanied and followed these critical experiences.

Many students did not have access to this kind of help when they encountered difficult conversations or intense grief-provoking experiences. Some were openly chastised for becoming personally involved with their patients when such incidents took place. Others became cautious in their conversational ventures because of conversational *faux pas* which occurred during the early weeks, when vulnerability to failure was acute. Still others felt guilty when they could not use the "right conversational techniques." As one put it,

> I was always in trouble. It came out, I ruined my process recordings and felt guilty. That was what it produced—a guilty feeling about what I was doing to the patients. . . . I would either come out with guilt feelings that I didn't use the tech-

11 Volkart has suggested that in American culture the role of the bereaved person, with its emphasis on loss, grief, and the open expression of these feelings, may be in conflict with the expected behaviors associated with other roles, e.g., the role of adult male. He adds further, "But to the extent that social and cultural conditions encourage interpersonal relationships in which overidentification, overdependence, sense of loss, hostility, guilt, and ambivalence are bred in profusion, and to the extent that the social role of the bereaved person does not take account of these feelings and the needs they inspire—to that extent bereaved persons may often be unintended victims of their sociocultural system." Edmund H. Volkart and Stanley T. Michael, "Bereavement and Mental Health," *Explorations in Social Psychiatry* (New York: Basic Books, 1957), p. 301.

niques, or I would come out with guilt feelings that I did use the technique but I didn't get anywhere, or I don't know what is going on really.

It is not surprising that the majority of students became skilled at avoiding conversations which offered more penalties than rewards, and more discomfort than satisfaction.

As this chapter has indicated, variations in awareness of dying, conversation under stress, and student experience play a major part in determining what happens to nurse students when they talk with dying patients. Both the conversational guidelines for providing psychological care and the anticipated results of such conversations are unclear to many students—thus they use their commonsense judgments in deciding what to say and when. In general, they learn many strategies for managing conversations which threaten to get out of control. They also learn ways of compensating for the helpless feelings which are engendered when they are assigned to dying patients. It is true that students have many positive experiences in talking with dying patients. It is also true that under some conditions the less positive conversational experiences can have far-reaching effects on the student, as a person and as a nurse. So also can assignments in which the student is brought into direct contact with death itself. The next chapter is concerned with the impact and aftermath of encounters with death.

Chapter 5 | Encounters
with
Death

For some students the first encounter with death may be remembered as a highly successful event. For others it takes place under circumstances so distressing that the student's memory is one of personal failure and horror. In either case it can leave a lasting impression by coloring the student's perspective on death in general, as well as by influencing the attitudes and behaviors that she will demonstrate whenever she meets it again as a nurse. This chapter describes the impact and meaning of encounters which are particularly significant to the students and delineates the circumstances under which memorable incidents take place. Students can encounter death in the hospital under many different circumstances. Some incidents make relatively little impression on the students, but others leave a lasting impression. There are two reasons why the incidents involving death tend to provide many significant experiences. First, death is an event with which most students are not very familiar, and second, these incidents often require some kind of performance by the student. Thus she has concerns and expectations about the adequacy of her actions. The results of encounters with death are often affected by one or both of these factors, the student's familiarity (or lack of familiarity) with death and the adequacy (or inadequacy) of her performance.

It is not death in the abstract which students encounter, but a complex situation with many different facets to which they can respond—a dead body, the hospital rituals used before and after death, the actions expected of nurses when they give physical care to dying patients, and the circumstances under which the death takes place. The context in which death occurs in the hospital is often a complicated one. The situation is further complicated by the fact that a student responds according to three different identities: as an individual, more or less familiar with death; as a nurse with obligations to fulfill; and as a student who may or may not have the encounter as part of a school assignment. Sometimes the student may be an observer only, or she may carry full responsibility as a nurse. The meaning of any given incident depends on what is happening and on the student's perception of her role (or roles) in it.

During the course of her life as a student, the nurse student may participate in one or in many incidents involving death. For many students the first encounter with death has singular importance. For one thing, many have not had personal contact with death, and have little concrete knowledge on which to base their expectations of what it will be like when encountered. First-time meetings introduce them to the unknowns of this important event. In addition, the students are concerned about how they will handle themselves, both personally and professionally, in the presence of death. Facing death successfully is viewed by them as a significant student experience. In consequence, the beginning student anticipates having this experience under conditions which will prepare her to cope with the nursing problems associated with it, and with herself.

I imagine that in medical surgical nursing we'll all be given the opportunity simply because it is part of it. In fact, I hope that I do have a chance because I think it would be better when I have people around. I'm not sure what my reactions will be, and as long as there are instructors and other people around who could help me work these things through, I think I would rather do it for the first time in nursing school, rather than have it happen when I'm a graduate nurse and there is no one really that I could talk with, as I could with instructors.

The students infrequently encounter death under the ideal conditions anticipated by this young woman.

The impact of many initial encounters with death comes about because the student is suddenly exposed to new and unfamiliar scenes. The impact is often intense because the act of dying in this society tends to produce strong feelings and discomforting behaviors in those who are involved with the dying patient, e.g., the family is often caught up in expressed and unexpressed feelings of grief and guilt, or the physicians are frustrated because their efforts—no matter how valiant—cannot prevent the patient from dying.[1] Dying is a hospital event with many tension-producing components, any one of which can precipitate strong feelings in the nurse student who does not anticipate these happenings. The student's perspective on incidents involving death can best be explained and understood when the circumstances surrounding death in the hospital are first clarified.

[1] When the social role in bereavement does not provide socially sanctioned outlets for expressing strong feelings, such as guilt or anger, the individual's behavior may exhibit signs of psychic stress—for example, a loss of emotional control, or stereotypical behavior in performing ordinary tasks. Some of the role conflicts and other psychological problems associated with bereavement and a social role preoccupied with the expression of grief are discussed by Edmund K. Volkart and Stanley T. Michael in "Bereavement and Mental Health," *Explorations in Social Psychiatry* (New York: Basic Books, 1957), pp. 296–301. Although it is not always clearly recognized, the hospital staff as well as the family are psychologically vulnerable to feelings of loss when a patient dies—thus defensive strategies develop to protect the staff from intense emotional involvement. See Barney G. Glaser and Anselm L. Strauss, *Awareness of Dying* (Chicago: Aldine, 1965), pp. 226–256.

Death in the Hospital

As an event normally a part of hospital life, the death of a patient is not an isolated episode but occurs as part of a sequence of events in which the patient, family members, and hospital personnel are engaged in various kinds of interaction.[2] What happens to these people—including nursing students—is determined by an interplay among several factors, especially the kind of death, the setting in which it happens, and the circumstances surrounding and leading up to the ending of the person's life.

Some Dimensions of Dying

In a hospital, as elsewhere, death can be sudden and completely unexpected, or it can come as no surprise. Spitzer and Folta have observed that hospital personnel perform with minimal confusion in managing the tasks associated with an expected death. When a death is unanticipated, interactions among the staff increase in frequency, and often the exchange of vital information takes place by unusual communication channels.[3]

A second important characteristic of death is that expectations about a given patient's death may be certain or uncertain. When death is certain, there are different anticipations and interactions than when death appears unlikely; therefore, the certainty-uncertainty dimension is an important one. A third important characteristic is the interval before dying: this may vary from a matter of minutes to weeks, and even years in rare instances. Differences in the length of time during which the patient is defined as dying set the stage for many different reactions and interactions which involve the hospital personnel, the patient, and his family. In some instances a patient is in and out of the hospital many times before his final stay, and the staff know him well, thereby increasing their vulnerability to personal involvement and grief when death finally comes.

[2] Glaser and Strauss, *ibid.*, discuss the complexities of these interactions.
[3] Stephan P. Spitzer and Jeanette R. Folta, "Death in the Hospital: A Problem for Study," *Nursing Forum*, Vol. 3, No. 4 (1964), pp. 85–92.

A fourth important influence is the mode of dying, the physical changes which occur in the dying person. These can have profound effects on him and on those around him. Depending on the cause, the dying process may bestow an easy death or, in sharp contrast, one difficult to endure and agonizing to behold. Death from an overdose of sleeping pills, for example, appears quite different from the end state precipitated by tetanus, as those who have seen both can testify. The impact of death can be conveyed not only through appearance, but also through stimulation of smell, hearing, or touch. Sometimes the sensory shock can be great. Thus it is difficult to block out the memory of the patient with smallpox, covered with unsightly pustules and surrounded by the fetid odor of infection. In addition, the death scene itself may appear almost dehumanized by all manner of technical equipment, grotesque in the impression it conveys to outsiders.

The actions and reactions of hospital personnel in response to a death are affected by the "death expectations" of the setting in which they work. In some wards where critically ill patients are present in large numbers, death may be almost an everyday occurrence, with well-formulated routines available for dealing with it. Intensive-care units and cancer wards are familiar examples of high mortality wards, though the dying process normally found in each may be quite different. In some parts of the hospital (and in some hospitals in general), death may be such a rare and disturbing phenomenon that personnel are little prepared to cope with it, and its occurrence takes them by surprise. Sometimes a patient dies in a setting where the event is even more completely unexpected, such as the waiting room of the X-ray department. Obviously the unexpected death can happen anywhere, but in the hospital certain types of death tend to be associated with certain ward settings. The emergency room deals with violent death brought in from the community. In the operating room a prearranged treatment may go awry and cause sudden death. In medical and surgical wards death not uncommonly appears after a progressive downhill course, which may be rapid or prolonged. A student can encounter death for the first time under any of these circumstances. In addition, there are other conditions which strongly affect the reactions she is likely to experience in response to a specific death.

Some Conditions Affecting Reactions to Death

An individual's reactions to a given death are influenced by many personal and social factors. As was indicated in the previous chapter, patients tend to be classified in terms of their values to society. The deaths of those with highly valued personal and social characteristics tend to produce grief and feelings of loss in everyone, perhaps most poignantly when those who die are children or young adults in the prime of life. In contrast, the demise of one with low social value may be practically unnoticed.

Personal impressions are also influenced by a patient's behavior in response to his dying. Individuals show wide differences in their styles of dying, and certain ways of behaving are more acceptable than others. From the hospital staff perspective, approval is generally given for being brave, for controlling a public demonstration of one's feelings, and for behaving with dignity or with humor. In contrast, staff endorsement is unlikely when the dying patient makes many demands for time and attention, or when he overtly expresses anger or criticizes their actions. Just as individuals behave differently while dying, so families can vary in their reactions to the death of one of their members. Some may present a stoic façade, whereas others may show an open and noisy display of grief, and some may not put in an appearance. Moreover, patients come from many different cultural and religious backgrounds with widely varying practices, beliefs, and sacred rituals associated with the dying process. These requirements influence the kinds of rites, personages, and behaviors associated with a particular death.[4] For these reasons the dying process is a social phenomenon with many variations. The differences create a variety of situations for hospital personnel to handle.

There are also many variations in what happens at the time of

---

[4] For a discussion of cultural differences as they influence patient expectations, see Esther Lucille Brown, *Newer Dimensions of Patient Care: Patients as People*, Part III (New York: Russell Sage Foundation, 1964).

death. The presence of persons at the final scene can vary greatly. Sometimes the patient dies alone and unattended. Sometimes family members are present, as is most likely when death is expected. On some occasions—as in emergency rooms—death is witnessed by many, including strangers as well as the hospital staff. In addition, there can be wide differences in the dying person's awareness of what is happening to him, and in the extent of open discussion which staff and family have allowed him. The person may be comatose, or he may be conscious and openly communicating until his final moments.

Death can also be described as a critical event which initiates change in two major ways. It interrupts whatever interaction or activity is in progress at that moment—whether this be watchful waiting, ongoing treatment, or social conversation. It provokes a response in those who are present, and each person reacts from his own perspective. The family may begin to grieve. The doctor may be concerned about getting permission for an autopsy. The nurse may wonder how other patients are going to take this news. The patient in the next bed may wonder if this will happen to him. In effect, each person responds to the situation in terms of its particular meanings to him, but these meanings are often divergent and lead to quite different perceptions and definitions of the situation. Because emotional tension is likely to be high at this critical time, the possibility is also high that those with different perspectives may misunderstand and misinterpret the actions of others.

It should be recognized that death is a task which American doctors and nurses find difficult to handle, both personally and professionally, even under the best of circumstances. As a result, they have developed many personal and institutionalized mechanisms for easing the strains of this work problem.[5] As persons to whom society has delegated life-saving responsibilities, physicians and nurses have a particular investment in preventing death. Thus their actions at the time of death (or in preventing death) carry

[5] Glaser and Strauss, *op. cit.*, pp. 177–225.

a special significance both to them and to those who are relying on their services. The meaning of their actions can easily be distorted by those who are personally involved with the patient's death.[6] As an inexperienced person, the beginning student can also interpret these actions through biased eyes. She tends to have unrealistic—sometimes highly idealistic—expectations about the behaviors of doctors and nurses when they are faced with saving a patient's life.

Fresh from the world outside, the nurse student is a stranger to the new sights and unfamiliar practices of hospital life. Moving from the protected position of outsider, she may have in the hospital her first exposure to the mysteries of death and to the rituals used in American hospitals for managing the situation. Initially she reacts to the unfamiliar scene, which includes how doctors and nurses behave around dying patients as well as how a dead body looks. What she sees often comes as a surprise, and sometimes brings disillusionment. She may also react to other aspects of this human problem, to the sadness provoked by an untimely death and to the loss experienced by a family.

As a person often inexperienced with death, she tends also to evaluate her own behavior in the situation and to judge herself on how well or how poorly she faces death as a human being. As a human being, she is also vulnerable to those psychological aspects which are personally meaningful, for the latter can still be present when death itself is no longer a novel experience. First encounters with death clearly demonstrate the impact that the dying situation makes on the uninitiated.

First Encounters and the Unfamiliar

Certain aspects of first encounters with death make an especially great impression. There are those associated with the mystery of death itself, and the dread surrounding this unknown but

[6] Erich Lindemann in "Symptomatology and Management of Acute Grief," *American Journal of Psychiatry*, 101 (September, 1944), p. 145, discusses these behavior patterns.

important life event. There are reactions in response to religious and hospital rituals and to activities going on around the dying person. There are also impressions which emerge when students confront the reality of medical and nursing practices and begin to give up their idealized notions about physicians and nurses.

The Mystery of Death

When students see death for the first time, they are aware of unexpected and varied reactions within themselves. First, there is the awesome, helpless feeling which takes place when one is in the presence of death. The living person who was there a moment ago is now gone. The inexperienced person undergoing this moment is deeply aware of the "thin line" between life and death, the mystic gap which separates the two. When a student is present during the transition period from life to death, she is likely to describe a mystical response, and a sense of wonderment and awe, and sometimes fear. By comparison, the student who enters the situation after the death has taken place—as happens to a student who unexpectedly finds a patient dead—talks of her surprise or shock at finding a body. The aura of mystery is missing.

Students are curious at first about the appearance of the dead. They do not know what to anticipate, and they often hesitate to "take a look" because they dread what they might find. Two aspects of appearance are prone to make an impression, the pre-death look of the dying person and the sight of the corpse itself. Some patients at the end of lengthy, disintegrating illness are emaciated and anguished in appearance, and students are amazed to see that they look better after they die. One young woman said, "Before she died, she was miserable looking and she had tubes in her nose. When I saw her about a half-hour after she died, she looked beautiful. It gives you a weird feeling to see someone die." Because many patients do not "look bad" during the process of dying, students also express surprise when they find that persons do not look much different when they are dead. Not all dead bodies look peaceful, of course, and a corpse which conveys the message of a *difficult death* strikes with great impact. A student whose first encounter was with a patient who hung himself will never forget the experience, nor will another whose first exposure was to a death following generalized septicemia. The appearance of the corpse immediately following death may resemble the living person but is quite different several hours later when color changes are well under way and rigor mortis is apparent. Students are often surprised by these alterations because they were not anticipated.

Of more concern than appearance of the corpse is the question of how it will feel. Sometimes students are able to view the dead body but avoid touching it, though they may want to do so. Those who touch a person who has just died are often surprised by the sensation they feel. One student commented, "I thought he would be warm, but I was surprised that he was warm." When a body is discolored or otherwise difficult to view, the student is even more reluctant to put her hands on it. As one said,

> Just within that five minutes the body began to change tremendously. It became all mottled, and very cold. I had not handled a dead body before, and it was all I could do to force myself to pick up the arms and collapse them over the front of the body so that they would not be hanging out. I then tried to shut the eyes because they were rolled back and very unnatural looking and rather disturbing.

The "dread about death" phenomenon is strongly reflected in the commonly expressed wish not to be left alone with the body.

Postmortem and Predying Rituals and Activities

Many first-time encounters introduce students to various hospital routines which come into play once a person has died. The students participate in such activities as preparing the body for removal to the hospital morgue and transporting it to that destination. Many are surprised to see how bodies are handled—for instance, they must be tagged for identification purposes; they are tied and wrapped for ease in transportation; they are removed to an icebox where they are kept until an autopsy is performed, or until the mortician removes them.

It is not the procedures alone which catch students off guard. More often the actions of hospital personnel are surprising, sometimes shocking. One student described these reactions,

> The way this orderly handled the body bothered me. I mean he was rough. They stripped the body down and tied the hands and legs together and kept the eyelids shut by putting pieces of cotton underneath them. Then he brought out a paper shroud and wrapped the body in that, covering the head. Then four of us picked up the body and put it on a tray and shoved it in the icebox. It was like putting a piece of meat in the icebox. I didn't like it at all.

When undergoing these experiences for the first time, many students are struck by the contrast between life and death. They are bothered by the impersonal or careless manners they see demonstrated as this rapid transition takes place. A student who had taken care of a patient prior to his death and then participated in taking his body to the morgue was struck by the disparity between the scene at his bedside with the "family there and so concerned and all" and the irreverent behaviors of the morgue attendants. In her words, "In nursing school we are taught to protect the body. When you think of banging a head, well, this just isn't done, but this seems to be nothing after death. We can do anything we want with the body." That the shift from person to body does precipitate a different focus was brought sharply home to another student who found herself, like everyone else, no longer referring to the person as "he" but as "it."

Depersonalization or joking behavior in the presence of death is extremely disturbing to the inexperienced student who has an image of physicians and nurses as concerned and professional in demeanor. Hence, one young student was frankly shocked when a resident physician stopped giving emergency care and began using the body to demonstrate procedures to some medical students. As she put it,

> After a few more minutes the one who seemed to be in charge decided to quit, that it was no use. It came to a very unspectacular end. At this point, I became more angry because the body of the patient turned one moment from a patient they were trying to save into a cadaver the next moment; they started to demonstrate to the medical students how to put in a trach tube, and this just annoyed me.

Although patients are often used for teaching purposes, this student was not emotionally prepared to witness such an abrupt shift from the practice of medicine to the use of a patient for medical student learning.

Just as depersonalized treatment of a person's body can disturb the inexperienced student, so can the expression of grim humor, an outlet which is often used by hospital staff to cope with their own discomfort.[7] The practical joke is a mechanism which often serves to relieve tensions, but humor in the presence of the dead can seem obscene to the idealistic newcomer. Moreover, teasing may not always achieve the desired effect and sometimes can provoke traumatic consequences. A young student who took a body to the morgue was locked in by her classmates as a joke. She has never forgotten the horror of the experience. Years later, as a practicing nurse, she has found it difficult to be around death and to participate in the care of dying patients.

Although students react at first to the use of grim humor by others, they also use joking to handle some of their own tensions. A student in her second year of school made these observations about a first-year student who had unexpectedly found a dead patient.

> Gee, I don't know how she felt. She was talking to another student and me about it. She was kind of making a joke about it. I don't know if she didn't realize everything that had hap-

---

[7] Renee C. Fox in *Experiment Perilous* (New York: Free Press, 1959), p. 231, points out that she became aware of the frequent use of "grim humor" as a tension release by both the patients and the physicians on a research ward when "I found myself in the act of making a macabre joke, and I can remember speculating on the source of my unlikely new talent."

pened or not. She said she just walked into the ward and to the door, and she could tell the patient was dead. She asked one of the orderlies to come in and look. He did, and they looked, and they went on about doing postmortem care. She didn't say too much about it except making more or less a joke about it.

Oh yes, first they called the doctor—that's kind of important. She didn't walk right in and—to me, she's kind of humorous. She knew the patient was dead and the orderly told her, "Go in and wake her up, shake her and wake her up." She went in and shook her, and she knew she was dead.

A problem the new student invariably finds troublesome is the prolonging or not prolonging of life when it is known that the patient will surely die. This question invariably arises when a student sees a patient kept alive by drugs and other miracles of modern medicine or, conversely, sees only minimal care provided. A young student described her reactions to the latter situation in this way.

I didn't even know she was dying. The doctor had taken these measures. As far as medical ethics are concerned, a doctor has to do for his patients only those things that are necessary to maintain life, nothing extra. In other words, there has to be a room where there is oxygen and a certain amount of food and a certain amount of fluid—that's just about all you have to do. This woman was 91, and it was my first experience with a spot where the doctor didn't have to put her in an oxygen tent even if she needed oxygen, and he didn't have to give her extra fluids although she was dying of dehydration.

I rebelled because I refused to care for her after that. I refused to even talk about it. There are several girls who agree with me, and there are several girls who thought it was right —she would never be any use to anyone. She would be a burden on society and her family couldn't afford to take care of her. Her hospital bill had run up into the thousands of dollars. The hospital couldn't care for her, and she would be an invalid. She had permanent damage as far as her mental abilities go. She would never speak again—the motor cells had been knocked out. I could see the reasoning there—she would be happier dead, but this idea of letting her die was something that I couldn't rationalize. It didn't fit in with my personality. Yet now I see how they could do it, but I still don't agree with it.

These experiences are disturbing to students because the practices carry moral and ethical implications, and students react to them primarily in terms of their own religious training and social background. That staff nurses have similar reactions to these problem situations is indeed true. The new and unexpected, however, carry a special poignancy for the uninitiated and stimulate many a dormitory discussion about the meaning of life.

First encounters with death and dying can introduce students to the unfamiliar in yet another way by exposing them to religious practices different from their own. Students report these rituals as "interesting," "surprising," and sometimes "upsetting." In describing her first experience with a dying patient, a first-year student was disturbed when the priest was called to perform the last rites of the Roman Catholic Church. In her words, "He was scaring her to death. Here he was saying the last rites and she wasn't going to die. Telling her nonverbally that your chances are pretty slim, and I thought she must be terrified, but I didn't say anything." Not only was this student unaware of the significance of extreme unction (anointing of those in danger of dying) in the life of a Catholic, she could not believe that the patient was dying and did not recognize the physical signs which forecast it. In a similar way, students can be upset when patients' religious or philosophical beliefs are at variance with their own. A student was frankly shocked when a patient dying of cancer scoffed at the notion of an afterlife and refused the services of a minister.

It is now readily apparent that the students have strong reactions whenever they encounter behavior which does not coincide with their expectations concerning what is "appropriate" in the presence of death. They are often surprised or shocked by the unanticipated actions of patients, their families, and the hospital staff as well.

Facing Reality: The Limits of Medical Practice

Inappropriate personal behavior in the presence of death is one matter. There are also other aspects of staff behavior which the students find troublesome. First, they must face the reality that physicians are not omnipotent and cannot save everyone. One student, who had listened to a group of physicians discussing the pros and cons of their management of a particular emergency, made this observation.

> The thing that struck me as a sign of weakness was the way they tried to reassure themselves that they had used the right choice of drugs. They were saying that, "It was right, wasn't it?" and, "Oh, yes, I'm sure that this was the correct choice." I knew that I could not help this patient, and if anybody could it had to be the doctors. I could not, at this time, tolerate their indecision and the feelings that perhaps they were not omnipotent.

Part of becoming a nurse is learning that doctors sometimes wonder if they have selected the best treatment, that doctors are human and subject to errors in judgment like all humans, but also that physicians are limited in their life-saving skills by the limits of medical science.

A second problem confronting new students is facing the fact that in the hospital world, as in all professional fields, there are practitioners whose performance is—or seems—poor or mediocre. As happens to all who enter a new career, first-hand experience brings surprise and disappointment, sometimes disillusionment, with the practices and behaviors of those whom the trainee has idealized. A young student who could not find a patient's pulse was terribly upset when the doctor did not rush to the bedside, at her request, but instead asked, "What service is he on?" Later she developed a different understanding of the doctor's position and of the pressures impinging on his time and energy. At that moment she expected him to drop everything and run. The most traumatic of such encounters are those in which the inexperienced student observes medical and nursing practices which frankly shock her. The brusque announcement to the patient, "You only have six months to live," or the intern's inability to perform cardiac massage expertly are upsetting to the student's notion of what a doctor *should be*. The staff nurse who ignored the brief respiratory efforts of a sixth-month premature infant and put it aside with the comment, "It won't live anyway," horrified the student, who was afraid to say anything at the time, yet has never forgotten the experience.

Just as students are disillusioned by some experiences, they are impressed and reassured by others. A student who watches a gentle staff nurse giving care to a terminally ill child is impressed by the sureness and comfort of this nurse's ministrations. The student who sees a physician bring sudden hemorrhage under control, or take time to explain a serious problem to the family, has a similar experience. It is apparent, however, that disturbing experiences stemming from the staff's inexpertness (apparent or real) carry an impact not easily forgotten.

Reactions to the Unfamiliar

Unfamiliar events can be disturbing, but they can also be exciting and stimulating. One student who was assigned to a dying patient regretted that he was her assignment because she had never seen anyone die. As she put it, "I wanted to be a spectator. I was curious about everything that was going on." Another student was aware that a patient in the ward (not assigned to her) had died because the doctors discontinued their efforts to resuscitate him. She commented,

> I went over to look at him after they left, and I assumed that he was dead. They didn't tell us, and the nurse said they should have, so that we would know if anybody did ask us. But I was really interested. We had been studying about the lungs, and I had an idea that something was wrong that would cause this labored breathing. It didn't bother me.

As a student she responded to this experience because it offered something to be learned, and she was curious. However, she showed her human responses when she talked about attending the autopsy.

> It is a cold room, down in the basement. I've walked by it many times now, and I cringe when I go by it. It is what you would picture as a morgue. It is cold, and you feel like you want to get out of there, if you can. I think the hardest part wasn't when he died. What bothered me was being *in that room* and realizing that that morning I had seen the man alive. Here he was dead now, and they were carving on him.

Attendance at an autopsy often makes such an impression, but students describe a range of reactions extending from "good learning experience" to "pretty ghastly." The difference often depends on the actions of the pathologist and the other persons in attendance, and the kind of atmosphere they create.

When students talk about their first experiences with death, they are sensitive to environmental details and very much aware of the people who are there. The presence of family members makes a great impression. One student assigned to a man in the final hours of his life referred to his family sitting outside the room as a "reminder." When asked, "Reminder of what?" she responded, "That the sick man was part of the family, and they were all sort of tall and wore dark blue suits, and they just sort of looked like undertakers. The woman was wearing a black hat with a veil and it just kind of suggested morbidity." This kind of sensitivity to detail is very much a part of first experiences with death. It is seldom present in the same clear way when students talk about their later encounters. Perhaps this sensitivity is a reflection of the significance which a first-time involvement with the ending of a life can carry, particularly in a society which protects its young people from direct participation in this aspect of human existence.

The Critical Importance of Unfamiliarity

Lack of familiarity with sickness and death and hospital life places the new student in an extremely vulnerable position because many events catch her off guard. In the beginning she is not particularly skilled at recognizing dying and often is not prepared for the possibility, even though the hospital staff is well aware of it. Even when she has been told, the inexperienced student tends to consider death as an unlikely possibility, as something which just doesn't happen to "my patients," and its coming takes her by surprise.

Beginning students are prime candidates for shock responses to the unexpected death. One first-year student described this reaction.

> He had had a convulsion that morning, and it was just the beginning of what you call the "dying part." I remember in team report the nurse telling me to be aware of convulsions, but I had never seen a convulsion before, and I didn't know what to look for and I asked. She said, "just when he would start shaking" and this started some anxiety in me because I didn't know whether I was capable of taking care of him or not, being so critically ill.

> Of course, he was in a room by himself, which meant that I would be in there alone without anybody else most of the time, and his family was there.

> That morning he started having convulsions, and I remember that I was in the room alone when he had one convulsion, and he started shaking, and I didn't know what was going on. I just stood there and watched him, and then I ran out to get my teacher, and I said, "He's shaking, and I don't know what's going on." So she ran back, and he had stopped and was just lying there.

> The wife was crying and was going in and out of the room, and the doctor had just told the wife that nothing more could be done, and she took this well at first, but then she did finally break down and she told her husband that things weren't quite as well as he made them out to be, and I just remember feeling so helpless. I did not know what to do. I was just standing there watching him die, and I think this hit me the hardest of all.

My teacher suggested that I give him a backrub so we started, and I don't think I will ever forget this. He stopped breathing, and she was rubbing his back. I was standing at the foot of the bed. All of a sudden you just didn't see his chest go up and down, and the son yelled out, "Oh, my God." He leaned down close to his father, and it seemed like forever, but it must have been only a minute. He took a great deep breath, and everybody just sort of sighed. The wife started to cry, and it just got too emotional, too heavy in the room, and I left the room and told my teacher that I didn't want to go in again.

It still scares me to see somebody, you know, one minute moving, and the next minute just lying there in bed like a vegetable.

Lack of experience makes the student susceptible to the impact of these unanticipated and emotionally unsettling events. It can also lead her into situations which wiser and more knowledgeable persons would avoid. The student who chose to go to the operating room with "her patient" was not prepared for the unforgettable picture of a child with half of his brain removed, nor could she understand why the doctors were performing the operation when they called the tumor "inoperable." She was not prepared for the unexpected visual trauma, and as an outsider, she had little awareness of privileged negotiations between the family and the doctor. When students are permitted and encouraged to choose their own experiences, they can get themselves into just such traumatic situations because they are ignorant of the possibilities which lie ahead.

Lack of experience also increases the likelihood of personal involvement with the death of a patient. Very often the initial encounter causes beginning students to think for the first time about the possibility of their parents' deaths. After her first experience, one girl reported these thoughts.

He was pretty sick when I was with him. Although one thing that I did do was kind of project a feeling and think about when my parents die. I think this played a big part. How are they going to treat them? This gets you all wrapped up in emotions.

Initially, students tend to become personally involved with their patients. The deaths of some patients, such as young children, lead to intense grief for which the student is not prepared. After a two-week assignment to a teenager who died, one student said that she could understand why the hospital personnel avoided these patients and kept themselves from being involved. Sometimes the involvement has a negative flavor. Thus the student can be disturbed by an assignment to a dying patient because she dislikes the patient. As one student said, "I think the woman had purposefully allowed herself to die because this type of acidosis can be cleared up in two or three days. It was her own attitude, and I didn't respect her." It is now easy to see how a lack of familiarity with the many tension-producing aspects of dying can cause a student to become upset or to get herself into an awkward or extremely disturbing position.

Unfamiliarity can also play a very important part when a student's actions or performance are at stake. In fact, some experiences can be traumatic because a student's lack of experience causes her to interpret her actions as negligent, even though no question of negligence is involved. A student's performance during an encounter with death (or near death) can be extremely meaningful to her—if she sees herself as *adequate* in what she does or, conversely, *inadequate* in her actions and decisions. There are several conditions which strongly affect the student's ability to perform in an adequate (or inadequate) manner, both as a nurse and as a student.

Adequate and Inadequate Performance

Some Conditions Affecting Performance

A student's capacity to perform in a *satisfactory* way—by her own and by others' standards—is determined to a great extent by her familiarity with what she is expected to do and by her ability to perform, with some degree of facility, the procedures and inter-personal interactions required by the assignment. Whether she can perform competently or incompetently while in an incident involving a patient's death usually depends on a combination of favorable or unfavorable circumstances. One important contributing factor is her state of awareness concerning the possibility that death will occur.

To know that a patient is going to die is a significant piece of information, and the timing of the death announcement (that is, when the student learns of the probability of death), as well as the circumstances under which it is delivered, cause different effects. When the student is told at the beginning of an assignment that the patient is dying, she has the advantage of being forewarned. She is thereby informationally prepared, though not necessarily emotionally prepared, should death take place while she is present or during the assigned period with a patient. Advance news can be protective in another way. The student has not yet come to know the patient and his family, and she may deliberately take steps to avoid personal involvement. When a student learns of an impending death after two weeks or more with a patient, she cannot so easily escape feelings of sadness and human concern. It is important to recognize that death and dying carry emotional overtones of great intensity. To know that a patient is going to die is unsettling information at best. To become aware of the possibility in the middle of an assignment can be an unnerving experience and can sometimes interfere with one's ability to use one's hands or to think clearly. Even under the best of circumstances students have difficulty in performing well when first assigned to terminally ill patients. They consistently report that they "feel and are disorganized," that the care takes longer than expected. Usually a student finds herself preoccupied with thoughts of the patient's forthcoming death. Conversation with the patient is sparse, and the student is engrossed in her own concerns.

A student's ability to perform satisfactorily is also affected by the amount and kind of rehearsal provided for the tasks required in the assignment. As was indicated in the previous chapter, inadequate rehearsal for conversations with dying patients leads to some serious consequences for the student; so also can inadequate rehearsal for the technical aspects of patient care. Satisfactory performance during assignments to terminally ill patients is related to rehearsal at two levels. First, the student has had some prior practice in performing the technical procedures expected of her. Second, she has been psychologically prepared to perform these tasks when the patient is known to be dying.

Most commonly psychological preparation for providing satisfactory physical care to those who are dying comes about through active participation in these assignments with someone who is relatively comfortable in the presence of death. A young nurse described two experiences which helped her in learning to handle her own feelings about death. During her first year in school she had an instructor who talked easily about death during classroom discussions. By her actions the teacher conveyed an image that death is a part of life—not something apart from it. The second positive experience took place shortly after this nurse had finished school. While engaged in her first job, she saw a staff nurse taking care of a dying patient in a very warm and natural way. It was a "wonderful opportunity to see someone act as though dying weren't something to run away from."

Finally, a student's performance when she encounters death is greatly affected by the actions of others, both her peers and those who represent authority. The latter play an important part in determining the outcomes of many encounters with death. Physicians, teachers, and the nursing staff are all in positions to offer approbation or disapproval. Their judgments and subsequent behaviors toward the student can sometimes make the difference between a positive and a negative experience.

There are two kinds of performance requirements, thus the students have two sets of concerns—those centering around adequate performance as a student and those concerned with proficiency as a nurse. Sometimes one or the other of these concerns is primary during a particular experience, but often both are operating to influence a student's perception of herself and her actions. Both she and other persons judge her performance as competent or incompetent on the basis of certain standards.

Competence: Nurse and Student Standards

Initially students are very concerned about whether they will perform well as nurses. They are afraid that they may not act appropriately when confronted with important nursing problems. This concern runs the gamut from inadequacy to negligence. (The absolute worst would be to kill a patient.) Students want to be adept at providing care and comfort, just as they want to perform well when faced with an emergency.

Certain problems concern all students and are particularly troublesome in the beginning. The students are concerned when they cannot use equipment, either because they do not know how or lack the needed skills. They are bothered because they are not sure of themselves in such matters as correct reading of the blood pressure, or being able to recognize the significance of certain physical signs. They have trouble giving injections which cause pain, and in moving patients who are in great pain. One student reported these reactions when she first encountered a patient suffering severe pain. "I asked her what the pain was like, and she told me that it was a sharp pain. I was afraid to touch her. I didn't want to precipitate this pain." When asked how she handled the assignment, the student responded,

> I was all thumbs and toes and everything trying to change this bed and give this bath. Every movement seemed to cause pain. She would grimace; she would clutch the side of the bed. It bothered me because I was hurting this woman, and I couldn't do anything about it. Also, she wouldn't talk. When I finally felt that I had to escape from the situation, I went out into the hall and felt that I was going to cry.

In addition to the technical difficulties they encounter, new students also find that doctors and nurses pay little attention to their words. Staff actions of this sort tend to confirm the students' feelings of uncertainty and inadequacy.

The concerns about adequate performance all become amplified when a student is assigned to a patient in the terminal stages of illness. Judgment as a nurse and skill in providing comfort have significant importance for the student at this time. There are several general areas in which the students want to perform with competence—the administration of delegated medical tasks, the provision of care and comfort for the patient, appropriate conversation or interaction with the patient, and appropriate conversation or interaction with his family. Depending on the circumstances a student can encounter success or failure in any or all of these areas.

In addition to competent performance as a nurse, the students also want to perform well as students. Some of the standards used for judging these activities were described in Chapter 2 in the section on "Student Accountability." The discussion there deals primarily with the expectations of teachers and others in authority and with the standards they establish relative to satisfactory performance. The students are also concerned about performing according to the expectations of their peers. In general, students are very supportive of another student who has an assignment in which a patient dies. One student made this observation.

> When I told my fellow students that I would be helping with some of the postmortem care, their reaction was, "If you need any help, let me know." This was a real big thing you know, and something that would be pretty hard. They expected that I might need help.

The students often show special concern for a classmate who is the first one assigned to a terminally ill patient.

> She's carrying the ball first. The rest of us come in contact with the natural apprehensions that patients have about their conditions. But other than that, we haven't had contact with anyone who might be a terminal patient.

The student herself wants to perform in a way which does credit both to herself and to her class. Thus she does not want to do anything which might be viewed as disgraceful—for instance, running away from a critical assignment, or losing self-control at an inappropriate moment.

Expectations and Concerns as Students

During an assignment to a patient known to be dying, a student can have doubts about her ability to provide comfort and care. As one student described it,

> I sort of had the feeling that this time I know what is going to happen in the end. I know that he will die, or we are reasonably sure. I think this is a great experience for learning—to go in and be with him. I find that I do doubt—the things that I do. I was thinking the other day that wouldn't it be better for this man to have someone more experienced in these things.

At the same time the student is also concerned about getting experience for herself. The student mentioned above continued by saying, "It might help him more, but then I thought—well, this is true, but you never learn by running away from it. You have to stay with it."

In general, the students do not want to lose control of their emotions when confronted with stressful situations. One student commented about the matter in this way.

> The instructors never once told us that we aren't supposed to cry, but we are supposed to control our emotions until we are away from the immediate situation—then afterward we can cry if we want to. I can't say that this is very easy to achieve.

They want to have experiences which "test" their abilities, yet often find themselves having difficulty when faced with the reality of distressing events. A student reported this experience.

> Two days later I found another patient dead, which was really something. I found the staff very helpful. When the one nurse told me to go ahead into the utility room, they didn't seem to look down on me because I was having a little problem with this—expecting it, getting used to it. They seemed to take it

matter-of-factly, which at the time I wasn't. Nothing was ever said afterward about my not taking my responsibilities after this person died, since he was my patient.

Despite the feelings of upset brought on by finding the body, the student thought of the experience as a positive one.

I was included in helping to support the family afterward. I wasn't pushed out because my first reactions were not of the most supporting nature. In other words, I felt that I was supported when I needed it, and yet after my immediate need had been fulfilled, I was included back on the same level as before. I thought this was good.

The nursing staff allowed the student to move out of her role as nurse long enough to regain composure, and then welcomed her back. For the student a critical test had been passed successfully.

The first person in a class to have an assignment involving death frequently becomes something of a celebrity—and even an authority. One girl reported this experience.

I talked to the rest of the girls, and my roommate. We were only six months through training. They were quite interested in what it was like and how I felt—mostly in how I felt. I think this has an awful lot to do with your whole religious upbringing and your own ideas about this.

Except in the beginning there is relatively little widespread communication among the students about their actual encounters with death and with dying patients. Thus the students often have difficulty in comparing notes about these critical incidents. Following her first experience in providing postmortem care, a junior student encountered a senior student in the elevator and commented, "Well, I had my first postmortem care today." At the time she felt somewhat awkward and thought to herself, "I wonder if she has ever done this." The senior responded by saying, "That must have been tough," but did not indicate whether or not she herself had had such an assignment.

The general lack of awareness among students about other students' experiences with death was the rule unless a student happened to be involved in a spectacular incident which was picked up by the student grapevine. In general, these incidents were traumatic experiences for the students directly involved in them, and also provoked a collective "traumatic response" in other students. Incidents which resulted in severe personal and collective reactions had a common characteristic, expectations of the assignment were beyond the student's ability to perform.

The Overwhelming Assignment

From the student perspective inadequate performance as a nurse takes place when the assignment responsibilities are greater than the student's abilities to meet them. These responsibilities may involve the provision of comfort care, the implementation of medical therapies, or interactions with patients and families. Frequently the overwhelming assignment involves a dying patient with many treatments and procedures in progress. As one student said about just such an assignment,

> I didn't seem able to function at all that morning. . . . I had suctioning, and I had never worked with oxygen before. I can remember how frightened I was of the equipment. When I counted the respiration, I didn't know whether they were going to stop.

In her second year, this student had never been assigned to a seriously ill patient before, let alone one near death. She felt personally inadequate because she was expected to perform procedures she had never seen demonstrated. She was intensely aware of the patient's labored breathing and ghastly looks, and of the family outside the door. She did not know how to answer the family's questions, and in her words, "I felt a great deal of responsibility toward them and toward her to give her at least good physical care. I felt inadequate to do any of them."

A similar experience happened when a dying patient was used for a student's first assignment in the hospital. In this instance the student did not know that the patient was dying, but she was unable to perform her assignment—taking vital signs—because the patient was antagonistic and rejecting. The unsteady fingers and trembling hands of the newcomer became worse under the strain of the patient's manner. The physical signs were difficult to read and record, and the inexpert student found herself panicked by her failure to find, let alone count, a weak and erratic pulse. To make matters worse, she was alone with the patient and got help with the assignment only when she ran out and got her instructor. In the opinion of the student, the assignment was "difficult because I was not sufficiently along in my awareness and knowledge to deal with the situation. I was unprepared."

The Satisfying Assignment

It can be readily seen that lack of familiarity with the tasks to be done, in combination with inadequate rehearsal, results in an overwhelming assignment, and usually in a traumatic experience for the student. Conversely, when the student has some knowledge of what lies ahead and receives help in performing the tasks to be done, she is likely to have an assignment remembered as both satisfactory and satisfying. A student who was assigned to catheterize a severely ill woman described what happened in this way.

> It had been a whole year since I had catheterized a patient, and I certainly wanted the experience. Miss Smith knew that I did. She stood there the entire time while I planned the procedure. I looked at her, and she nodded "yes" or "no," or she gave me very direct hints as to how I could do this a better way. I think the whole thing just went beautifully.

When unfamiliarity is replaced by explicit direction and when a supporting environment is provided, the assignment tends to provide positive outcomes for the student.

Even under the best of assignment conditions, errors in judgment or procedure can sometimes occur. In the student's view negligence is *the most serious offense*. Students dread the thought of making serious mistakes or of harming patients by inadequate or negligent performance.

Making a Mistake

In carrying out delegated medical activities—most commonly the giving of medications—there is always the possibility of making a mistake. With the beginning student this is likely if supervision is minimal; with the older student it takes place because of carelessness or because of work pressures. In either case the experience is an upsetting one. A senior student who accidentally gave a patient the wrong drug made this observation.

> Luckily it was discovered. I don't know what I would have done if it wasn't. The patient was taken to emergency and his stomach was pumped out. It was quite a learning experience. . . . I almost quit school, I was so upset about it.

If self-accusation is reinforced by accusation by others—the physician, the teacher or supervisor, or the family—the situation is even worse for the student to bear. In this instance, however, the student reported, "I was harder on myself than those above me were."

Sometimes a treatment order by the physician produces an untoward effect, and the inexperienced student can blame herself. One girl told this story.

> I had a patient to whom I gave demerol. She had a bone marrow study, a sternal puncture, right after. After the procedure she began to go into shock and get progressively worse, and I began to work with her. The next day I came on only to discover she had died the evening before. I had not anticipated this death. This was not a critically ill patient but a diagnostic procedure, but I discovered that this was no small traumatic experience.

When she learned of the death, the student thought, "Did I kill the patient?" Being told, after the fact, that the patient had a poor prognosis did not completely erase the terrible feelings this particular death announcement carried.

Making a mistake, or believing that one has made a mistake, which does injury to a patient is a serious matter for the student involved. Thus, it can readily be understood that students are concerned about avoiding errors in performing procedural tasks. So also are they concerned about avoiding interactional errors with patients and their families. In managing the interpersonal aspects of assignments to dying patients, the students are likely to encounter difficulties they had not anticipated.

Inadequacy in Patient-Family Interaction

The students want to be successful in their conversations with patients. They can feel inadequate when they are prevented from achieving this aim because the patient is "difficult" or wants to talk about upsetting topics. In a similar way, beginning students find themselves inadequate when assigned to nonresponsive patients. The students wonder whether or not to engage in conversation, as they have been told by their teachers is the right thing to do. The comatose patient with staring eyes can be disturbing to see. Carrying on a conversation with this person seems unreal and awkward. Students who make the effort to talk to comatose patients are sometimes subjected to hazing by the staff. One student reported that a staff nurse walked to such a patient's bedside and commented disparagingly to her, "Oh, he cannot hear you. He's too far gone."

Just as they want to be effective with patients, so do students want to manage their interactions with family members in a proficient and appropriate way. The students often do not know how to cope with the family of a patient who is near death. A student offered this observation about one of her assignments.

> It wasn't so bad because I was trying to look at everything objectively, and I hadn't known this patient. I didn't get a chance to know her personally or to become involved with her because she was almost semiconscious. The thing that really bothered me, I guess, was the family—trying to give support to them in an empathetic way.

In this incident the student felt inadequate because she did not know how to provide support. Some interactions with families precipitate difficulties *because of* the student's actions. Inadvertently she may say or do something which backfires and causes her to blame herself, as the following incident illustrates.

I had been caring for the patient for two days. The wife asked me about 10:00 if she could leave for a couple of hours, and I told her I thought so. I didn't think anything would happen. Just as I was walking to the Nurses Station (after having found the man dead) the wife came back and, I don't know—perhaps the expression on my face—but she started hollering, "Oh, he's dying; he's dead." I didn't know exactly what to do so I went in and got the doctor, and I took the wife and talked to her. For a half-hour they tried to revive him and it just didn't work, and the wife and daughter were both there. That was the hardest for me because I had told the wife that I thought it would be all right. I know you can't say when a person is going to die, but it was the look on her face. And I had told her that I thought it would be all right.

In this instance the student felt inadequate because she had misled the family, "But I had told the wife, and this hurt me because I felt—well, I knew I shouldn't tell her when he was going to die, but I just didn't think it would be that soon." Students can have similar feelings of inadequacy when they say or do something which causes someone in the family to burst into tears or become very angry.

Generally speaking, the students felt helpless and inadequate when families became very upset or demanded special attention. Some students talked about helping families to grieve, but did not always know *how* to accomplish the task. A student's sense of inadequacy and helplessness clearly shows in this incident.

A nurse told me to talk to a particular wife. She had been out there talking to her—this woman whose husband had died. She said, "Would you walk Mrs. So-and-So and go to the chapel and sit with her for a while." This was a first for me.

I didn't know what to do, so I went to the chapel to sit with her. I didn't know what to say, but she didn't talk—she just cried. I told her that I hoped she had found out—well that maybe this would be a better place for her to sit right now, and I would get her the minister. I asked her if she wanted me to stay there longer, and she said that she would be all right.

The students found few explicit guidelines for managing interactions with families of dying patients, and their commonsense decisions about what to do sometimes got them into personal difficulties. For one thing, they found that conversing regularly with the family often caused them to become personally involved with them, and with the patient. In many ways the students found dealing with the dying patient's family a very distressing and difficult, and not always personally rewarding, task. When the instructional program emphasized the importance of psychological care for patients and their families, the students were prone to feel even more inadequate because they "should" provide something.[8]

Adequacy in Interactions with Families

As was indicated in the previous chapter, students can sometimes compensate for their helpless feelings about a dying patient by providing support for his family. Sometimes the student simply serves as a sounding board.

I talked with the wife quite a bit. This is another place where support is needed, and I feel I can give it sometimes. She feels

[8] The students who graduated in 1963 from the undergraduate program of the university school of nursing reported dealing with the family of a dying patient to be more upsetting at the time of graduation than was anticipated at the time of entry into the school. In a group of twenty-seven students, at entry 19 per cent anticipated that dealing with the dying patient's family would be highly upsetting, whereas at graduation 54 per cent of the same group reported the actual experience as highly upsetting. (This analysis was limited to students who actually encountered the event.) These data were provided by the Nursing Careers Project (USPHS Grant NU 00024), School of Nursing, University of California, San Francisco Medical Center. Staff members: Fred Davis, Virginia Olesen, Elvi Whittaker.

that when he does die, she will probably just fall apart; therefore she's made as many arrangements as possible beforehand. She's doing very well. She also likes to talk about just anything—little things that happened in her lifetime. I feel this is one way I can help her.

Sometimes she provides a family member with the needed chance to express his grief.

The evening that she died—she was calling out to God to let her die—her mother just went over in a corner and broke down. I felt that I was giving moral support to the mother at this time. You know, I really felt strongly about it—you know, if this were my child, I know that I would react in the same way. But later that night when she did die, the mother didn't cry. She had really done all of her grief work that evening when I had been with her.

Students who accept the concept of helping patients and families to engage in "grief work" are gratified when their efforts to provide support achieve some visible results.

I knew that the mother was going to have to talk about it. I knew she was going to have to express her fears. The mother mentioned to me several times that she was just fine until I came, and then she would start crying.

I thought that this was good for her. She had to go through this. I really think that my role at this time was quite vital to her because she had completely refrained from relating to the medical staff. She became very stoic in her conversation with everyone else. In fact, she even said that the reason that she did cry around me was that she trusted me and that she knew I understood. I told her that it was good for her to cry and talk about this.

Finally, the students can get a feeling of adequacy when they involve the family in providing physical care for the person who is dying.[9]

---

[9] Glaser and Strauss, op. cit., pp. 164–167, discuss "the relative as worker."

An assignment to a dying patient is important because the student wants to perform well in her own eyes. She achieves personal gratification when she does so. However, she also wants to meet the teacher's expectations for completing the assignment satisfactorily.

Meeting the Teacher's Expectations

Often successful completion of an assignment as a "good nurse" will be equivalent to being a "good student." However, an inability to complete the assigned tasks—particularly when other patients are involved—can raise questions in a student's mind about her competence.

> I knew that I had another patient to do, and all this time I had this real frustration feeling. I knew that there were a few things that needed to be done, for instance, the dressings to be changed. But I knew that everything that I did on him took away time on my other patient, who is going to be living and has a good prognosis.

The student thought she had handled the assignment pretty well, and found her teacher agreeing.

> I don't think that I did too badly on it. My instructor said that she thought I gave the patient good care. I don't know if she thought I needed moral support or what. I do feel that I did give him good care. I feel that where I lacked was in giving my other patients care.

This kind of reassurance, that one is performing in a satisfactory way, gives the student a sense of support and encouragement. Conversation of this sort also lets her know whether or not her standards and the teacher's standards are similar.

Sometimes students find that their standards for care are at variance with the standards imposed by those in authority. In the incident described on page 135, the student left the room because she was disturbed by a patient's intense pain made worse by her actions. The student talked to her teacher about her concerns.

She wanted to know what was the matter. I said that this woman is in pain, and I am causing more pain rather than alleviating it. My instructor said, "That is unfortunate but, you know, she can't have the pain medication every hour, and certain things have to be done." Well, I fiddled around and did just about anything I could to avoid doing anything more to this woman until such time as I could give her a pain medication, but I did have to have that bed changed and that bath given, although I refused to do her back.

Describing what took place later in the day, the student reported,

Later in conference I was very angry when the instructor all of a sudden miraculously said, "Well, why did you feel it necessary to give this bath and do these procedures when the patient was in pain? Wouldn't it have been better for you to wait until after you had given the pain medication?"

I was angry because I was caught in a web of circumstances. I had the authority of my instructor telling me what I had to do, and my inner voice saying not to do it. I had a patient who I was unable to help so I felt useless and incompetent, which increased my anxiety for wanting to disobey the instructor. So I ended up being rather ineffectual because my own level of anxiety interfered with my functioning.

An inability to complete the assigned tasks can bring an overwhelming sense of inadequacy as a student. The feelings of personal deficiency generated during the assignment can be enhanced or diminished by the actions and demeanor of the teacher or supervisor. That a difficult assignment can be made additionally difficult by a teacher is illustrated in this description of the first day of an assignment to a dying patient.

I remember that it was very hectic. I felt very inadequate, very stupid, very unable to handle it. I asked my instructor questions. Whenever I did, I got answers that made me feel foolish and childish for even approaching her.

At the end of six days, the student described the assignment as "one bad experience." In fact, she dreaded ever working in that part of the hospital.

There are other teachers who recognize the tensions and strains when students are assigned to perform tasks which are new and unsettling. A student made this observation about the help she received when assigned to provide postmortem body care for the first time.

> Her whole attitude, I think, formed my attitude of how to care for these people. She was very respectful and bathed him and, you know, didn't make any jokes about it. It was done seriously, and yet with due respect. I wasn't frightened anymore. I just realized then what death was—I saw here that the body's life had gone now.

Sometimes the teacher's presence and approach in working with the student can provide both direction and encouragement. As one student put it,

> I never interpreted their presence as being overpowering, or as the real authoritative figure in the presence of the patient. I mean, it is understood naturally that the instructor knows more than you do. I think that these particular instructors are very considerate of this—of the student nurse's position. They give all respect to the student nurse, in front of the patient. I see their presence as assistance, much more than actually taking over.

To judge from the experiences described by students, many teachers do not recognize the pressures they are exerting on students who are already feeling overwhelmed by the presence of death and by their own incompetence. The teacher's failure to recognize the serious import of these experiences can result in a student being sent alone to perform postmortem body care for the first time, or being forced to complete a distressing assignment with little assistance or support. The situation is even worse, of course, if the student gets a poor grade for the assignment or fails the course.

From a performance viewpoint the student has three basic concerns when she is assigned to a dying patient. She does not want to be inadequate or negligent as a nurse. She wants to perform well as a student. She wants to help the patient and his family. To experience failure on all three simultaneously is a devastating personal experience, and the dying patient can be a hazardous enterprise for those who are both inexperienced and unprepared.

Some Changes in Perspective Through Time

Difficulties with providing comfort and care for dying patients (as well as for other patients) decrease as skills are gained, more opportunity is provided for shared responsibility, and familiarity with the management of hospital work is gained. Paradoxically, the new student is vulnerable to terminal-care assignments because she lacks experience, whereas the more advanced student becomes vulnerable because, in her own eyes, she is "supposed to know the basic skills" of nursing. Whereas the beginning student can use the teacher's "failure" to explain her own inability to cope with a nursing problem, the older student finds this mechanism less acceptable and is more prone to blame herself. The senior, far more than the first-year student, expects herself to perform well not only with routine tasks but also in an emergency. Faced with her first heroic situation, the senior is extremely vulnerable to self-accusation if she does not handle the problem well, by her own standards. Obviously if she has had prior experience with hospital crises, she is better prepared for meeting these contingencies.

It has already been shown that dying is a hospital event with many tension-producing components. Any of these may produce strong emotional reactions in a nurse student. Not all encounters with death or dying cause intense reactions, however, but they are likely to do so when one of the following situations prevails: (1) the student becomes personally involved in the patient's death, or with the family; (2) the student is shocked, perhaps acutely traumatized, by some aspect of the death itself; (3) the student comes through the experience with strongly positive or negative feelings about how she handled herself in meeting the situation. There are several conditions which maximize the chances that students will react strongly during assignments to dying patients.

Reactions to Death and Dying

Conditions Contributing to Positive and Negative Outcomes

How a student reacts to a given incident involving death depends on a patterning of circumstances, and some events make relatively little impact because the conditions under which they take place carry little emotional weight. It has already been shown that awareness concerning the possibility that death might occur is one factor critically affecting the student's reactions to an assignment.

Lack of awareness of impending death is a condition which increases the possibility of a shock response should death unexpectedly take place. There are other circumstances which maximize the possibility that a given experience will be upsetting. The student is present when a patient dies unexpectedly. The death itself is difficult to watch, or the patient's style of dying is distressing to see. The possibility of negligence, by the student or by others, is associated with the death. The hospital staff or the family behave in unexpected, usually disturbing, ways before or at the time of death. The student receives open disapproval or an accusation of negligence from the family or from the staff. The student has little personal support both during and after the experience. One condition alone may not bring an untoward response if there are other circumstances which counterbalance the upsetting aspects of the situation, but there are times when one condition can be sufficiently significant to provoke severe psychological distress. When two or more of these conditions combine in a single incident, the possibility of upset increases accordingly.

Students react to some deaths not because of shock or surprise but because of personal involvement with the patient or the family. Personal involvement is maximized under the following conditions: (1) a lengthy assignment or prolonged contact with the patient; (2) an assignment consisting of only one or two patients; (3) a high social-loss patient; or (4) a personal friend as a patient. Personal involvement is minimized under the following circumstances: (1) a short assignment; (2) patient assignment as hospital work—multiple patients; (3) a low social-loss patient.

Just as some conditions are inclined to cause upsetting situations for students, other circumstances are conducive to positive experiences. The student is aware in advance of the possibility of death. The mode and style of dying are easy to watch and to manage. The family behaves in a manner that is not disturbing. The assignment has a limited duration. The student feels supported throughout and after the experience. Hospital staff behave in accordance with the student's expectations of appropriate behavior. The student performs well by her own criteria, and may also receive approval from significant others.

A student's ability to function effectively—both as a student and as a nurse—can be markedly affected by the intensity of her reactions to the death of a patient. Without quite knowing how it came about, some students find themselves living the role of bereaved person.

Grief and Bereavement

When students are first assigned to dying patients, they do not anticipate the reactions which will take place when the patient dies. One student put it this way. "I didn't realize at all how attached I had become to him because there was nothing—it wasn't anything you noticed. It was just little ways, you know." To her surprise she had trouble in realizing that he was dead. "For a couple of days after that, I found myself in the evening thinking, 'I must remember to tell Mr. So-and-so; he will be interested,' and then I think, 'no, he isn't there anymore.'"

Just as family members can have guilt feelings as well as feelings of loss when a patient dies, so also can a student.

She was a hard patient to take care of, and I knew she was going to die. I liked her a lot—I really did, but she was a hard patient to take care of. I thought, "I'll try to do as much for her as I can." Then after she did die, I thought, "You know —that there were a lot of times when I could have been nicer to her." Maybe it wouldn't have been better for her, but she was dying—and what was more important, making her feel good, or getting some little petty thing done.

Under some conditions, a student can also be glad when death finally comes.

I guess it was the last, or maybe it was the second to the last day, I really can't remember exactly, but in the last week she was still ambulatory but progressively got weaker and weaker, just extremely so. When I saw her crawling on her hands and knees and asking for pain medication and then after she had been given some, I finally realized that here I had done everything to keep this woman alive and felt that this woman should stay alive as long as she could. It really affected me and I— well, this woman wants to die, and why shouldn't she. She is about to die. Why should she have to go through this.

The intensity of a student's grieving is directly related to the degree of involvement with the patient and his family. One student described her reactions in this way.

The first night I didn't cry, except that I did call my roommate on the phone. I found that I couldn't talk, but that was the only time that I really started to cry. I found that I really never did cry, throughout the whole weekend, except that I became extremely snappy and irritable, and I did start to cry a lot of times.

Another student found herself playing the role of bereaved person with the patient's family.

She reminded me of my mother, sort of. She just was a lovely person. She talked about her home, and the things they used to do together, and a little bit about their financial status. Then the night that he died, I went over. It was a Sunday night. I went over in my lab coat to help a little bit. He died early the next morning so I didn't see him die, but she told me that night that when this is all over, "I'm going to come back and see you girls," and she did.

She came back last week and brought us some gifts. We both became upset but it wasn't uncomfortable because I think we both had established a relationship with each other too.

Another student found that her role as nurse served as a counterbalance for her feelings of intense concern and personal involvement.

I was extremely concerned. I feel that I was just kind of grasping with her to tell you the truth. I think one thing that really kept me going was the fact that I did know the situation better than she did. In my role as a nurse, I think that —it is hard to explain.

She then went on to explain that by being in a supporting role with the patient, she was able to attenuate her personal concerns.

A student can become so involved in grieving that she manifests the somatic and psychological symptoms described by Lindemann.[10] Sometimes these reactions are so intense that the student is unable to function according to the expectations of the teacher. A student, who had been intensely involved with a patient at the end of one semester, found herself doing "D" work at the beginning of the following semester. She said that she was "preoccupied with thoughts" about the previous experience. Her new teacher, however, did not appreciate the "absent-minded" behaviors and commented, "She hasn't even been trying. I just told her that it made me mad when someone with ability didn't use it." The teacher was not aware that the student's limited ability to function effectively was a function of a "terribly involving kind of experience." Because the student is accountable to the teacher (or the hospital staff) for performing adequately, the student can suffer secondary effects from intense grief reactions which prevent her from completing assignments in a satisfactory way.

[10] Lindemann, *op. cit.*, p. 141.

The Significance of Unassigned Events

When students are assigned to dying patients, they are held accountable for certain events deemed important either by their teachers or by the hospital staff. In implementing the assignments, however, the students constantly encounter many *unassigned events* which are also part of the context. No doubt the work day of the nurse student is filled with countless of these unassigned events, most of which are quickly forgotten along with the patient. Interviews with students indicate that the unassigned events are the salient ones in their memories, whether pleasant or unpleasant, of significant death encounters.[11]

Not all encounters with death are significant. Many are rapidly lost because the impression they leave is minimal, or the student has had so many experiences that she becomes relatively immune to the impact. When the unassigned events combine in certain patterns, they lead to important memories: those which are described as "good," as a "challenge," or as providing a sense of "accomplishment," and those which fall into the category of "awful."

Memories of the Good Experience

The term *challenge* is used to describe an incident in which a student lives up to her highest expectations and performs well. A sense of achievement can come from a "care and comfort till death" assignment or successful performance in an emergency. In either case, it is an assignment she is able to handle well, and she comes through the experience with an awareness of personal adequacy. What is also important, the student does not see herself as having been left alone to cope with a difficult problem, although sometimes the "support" comes afterward. In fact, handling an emergency alone is a greater achievement than meeting a heroic situation with a team, but the former can easily

11 Jeanne C. Quint, "The Hidden Hazards in Patient Assignments," *Nursing Outlook*, 13 (November, 1965), pp. 50–54.

become a failure if the student does something wrong and has no one with whom to share the responsibility. The student's memory of successful performance in an emergency is enhanced if she also receives commendation from the staff, thus obtaining recognition from others as well as from herself. Furthermore, recognition by the teacher can make the event even more important by incorporating success as a student into the final picture. However, many emergency incidents occur when the teachers are not present, and the students may not even report the incidents.

Accomplishment rather than *challenge* is the word most commonly used to describe a successful first-time experience in performing terminal-care activities associated with the expected death. Unlike the emergency situation, support in this instance means sharing the work experience with someone who is understanding and helpful. Thus whatever difficulties or surprises are encountered, they are counterbalanced by the availability of someone who comes through as needed. The teacher does not leave the new student with a patient who is about to expire. The aide quietly explains postmortem body care to the young student as they complete the assignment together. In effect, the student does not face the strain alone. Often these incidents take place when there is minimal involvement with the patient or his family, either because of limited contact or because the death is viewed as a welcome one. One student described her first experience in this way.

> I knew that he was going to die; everyone knew this. The family knew it. The wife had requested that he not be prolonged, that he be allowed to die comfortably. She did not want IVs started; she did not want all those other things going on. I had taken care of him for some time in the past, and I had gradually seen his progression to his death. By the time he died, I was quite willing to see him go, because you could see that he had lost all of his lifelike qualities, shall we say. He was comatose before his death, and it was something he went through peacefully. It was not a nerve-wracking experi-

ence. . . . Actually preparing the body really was not traumatic, and I didn't feel it, yet I thought about him a number of times afterwards. I didn't feel any great emotional effect. I had accepted that this was going to happen. He was in his seventies, which was not perhaps as bad as it would be for a young person to die.

This incident especially highlights those properties which maximize the possibility of a sense of accomplishment in giving terminal care—a peaceful death, low social loss, a gracious family style, dignified professional behavior, and an open awareness of impending death.

Memories of Difficult Encounters with Death

Students are upset by incidents in which they perform inadequately or make mistakes—the more serious the error, the more likely that the student will be deeply affected. Whenever a patient dies and a student attaches a cause-and-effect association between her actions and that death, the incident is traumatic for her. Sometimes, however, students have painful memories less because of "responsibility" than because something in the encounter is striking or shocking or personally meaningful. A student may remember a death which was "terribly sad" because she knew the patient personally, or responded to feelings generated by the high social loss he represented. The death of any young adult with a promising career is likely to bring forth this response—often a collective one also shared by the hospital staff. Sometimes a death is upsetting because the student is sensitive to, or involved with, the family. She may weep more for the mother who has lost her baby than for the death of the infant— that is, she may actively participate in grieving because her involvement is associated with significant personal meanings.

Some memories remain vivid because of events which trigger a shock reaction; thus it is not surprising that students remember unexpected deaths, or horrible deaths, or experiences which appear grotesque and obscene. If a given incident contains several shocking conditions, the student's upset is correspondingly increased. When both shock and personal involvement are present, the probability is even greater that the patient's death will be personally upsetting. For example, a student often is disturbed by the unexpected death of a patient whom she likes, but the experience can be worse if she is the person who finds the body.

By far the most traumatic memories are those in which horror, personal involvement, and negligence are combined in one incident. It is just such experiences which provoke this kind of comment. "You know, I worked as an aide before, and I've seen kids die before, but I have never been involved like this. I've never felt this way, and I never want another one like this." This student was assigned to a twelve-year-old boy with an inoperable tumor, and she became personally involved for several reasons. She had picked this assignment because she knew it was a terminal case, and she wanted to do a nursing study—but many things happened that she did not anticipate. The parents had lied to the child about never having surgery again, and this bothered her. The surgeons had decided to operate on an "inoperable" tumor, and she could not understand why. The boy had actively withdrawn from conversation with anyone, including her, when his parents told him of the impending surgery. In her intense concern for this youngster, the student accompanied him to the operating room where she was additionally upset by the "crass behavior" of the surgeons, by the bloodiness of the operation, and ultimately by the unexpected death on the table (unexpected, at least, to the student). When she returned to the ward and tried to talk about these upsetting matters, the nurse in charge commented, "Well, what do you expect? You're a glutton for punishment." This situation was further complicated by the student's question as to whether or not she had helped the boy. This concern was uppermost in her mind because the teacher had held a ward conference on "helping patients to die," on the day prior to this incident. During the week which followed, the student had terrible dreams and often talked in her sleep. One night her roommate woke her to ask, "Did you think you had killed him?"

The importance of this incident is that it illustrates the serious consequences which follow when the right combination of circumstances is present—in this instance, high social loss; an unexpected death; a distasteful death to see; an unacceptable family style; active rejection by the patient; personal involvement with the patient, and a concern about the actions of others toward him; inappropriate behaviors by doctors and nurses; the question of personal adequacy, perhaps negligence, as a nurse; and inability to complete a school assignment satisfactorily.

Whenever a student finds herself unable to cope with an assignment, as in the preceding incident, she generally seeks for help—and does this in two ways. She wants assistance in deciding what to do and in implementing the decisions that are made. She looks also for help in handling her own feelings. Some potentially traumatic incidents are attenuated because a sensitive teacher moves in, or a staff nurse takes over principal responsibility, when a student asks for help. In contrast, some incidents become worse because the teachers or the staff do not recognize the student's deep concern and fear. They chastise her instead of offering assistance. Indeed, some students are handicapped by a teacher's stereotyped expectation that they "should be" able to handle dying patient assignments. Students who are older when they entered nursing school are likely to be judged in this way, although not always correctly. Some teachers do not offer them the close supervision and support that they give to younger members of the class. Such a student may stumble through a difficult assignment, but the trauma remains long afterward. Thus a teacher's erroneous assumption of a student's previous experience and potential ability can lead to unfortunate consequences.

The Aftermath of Encounters with Death

The death of a patient is a serious matter. Although from the nurse and student perspectives "nothing more can be done" to help this person recover, from the human perspective encounters with death tend to provoke reactions which are personally disturbing. These events serve as reminders of the limits of human existence. As one student wrote,

> Life is my right to be transported by the sight of a wisp of a cloud traveling through the blue sky, to feel the cool, crisp breeze on my eyelids and cheeks, to experience sadness and joy. At this time I want to live, to feel, to perceive with every fiber of my body alert to this purpose. Death provides the meaning for life, but at this time in my life I cannot accept the concept of a close future death. I rebel and fight against it with the same energy which I direct into my method of living. Death verifies life, makes life too precious to relinquish it easily.

That encounters with dying patients precipitate thoughts about personal death, as well as philosophical discussions about it, is supported by the students' reports of their reactions following significant and meaningful experiences. Thinking about one's own dying is very threatening to many. Not surprisingly, the feelings and ideas engendered by their initial encounters with death threaten and upset the students. As a result, some learn to minimize their contacts with dying patients—and thereby keep themselves essentially protected from contemplating their own fears about death.

When they took part in meaningful incidents involving death, most students described needs to talk about their experiences. If the experience was a highly positive one, the student usually felt exhilarated and anxious to share what had happened. When the incident was a serious or traumatic one, students described a somewhat different pattern—with immediate and delayed responses. Immediately following the latter type of experience, some students did not want to talk. They reported that they could not concentrate in class, and they were constantly preoccupied with the events which had transpired. Some students feel "down" or "depressed" for the remainder of the day following an unsettling experience. Sometimes classmates or teachers tried to force the student to talk about the incident in a ward conference.

Students in this frame of mind reacted to this encroachment on their privacy as a "lack of understanding and sensitivity." In other instances, students were ready to talk because the timing of the conference was in tune with a state of readiness, and these students used the class session to ventilate their concerns and thereby to release some of the tension. The more serious the incident, however, the more likely it is that a student will seek counsel from *one* highly selected individual and will pull away from a group discussion of the incident—at least until the initial impact has been countered.

Immediately following an extremely traumatic experience, a student may describe herself as "in shock" for two or three days before she can begin to let down. Another can talk during this period to a trusted confidante, and only after she has "talked things out" does she find other feelings emerging. It took two days for one student to feel twinges of guilt because, "I didn't feel I had done a good job." Most of these students found their listeners outside the teaching staff, but a few students did turn to teachers whom they could trust. In general, roommates or close friends bore the brunt of listening, although husbands and boyfriends got their share. A few students sought guidance from the clergy, and some turned to their families. Following an extremely distressing assignment, one student made a cross-country telephone call—in search of support from her parents.

From the student perspective, talking about such incidents serves two purposes. The student is able to clarify her thoughts about the incident by relaying it to another person. The process also enables her to understand somewhat better her own feelings and reactions to the experience, and toward the other people involved in it. Often a student reported that she needed to talk more than once during the next two or three weeks, and periodically she would find herself reminiscing about the incident. Some students found little opportunity to talk about their experiences because they could not find people who would or could listen. Listening is not always easy, as is shown in this comment by a student.

While we were in obstetrics, one of my roommates was in pediatrics. She worked with a family of a little girl who failed cardiac surgery. She had prepared them, even knowing the possible outcome, for a hopeful outcome. She felt hopeful about it. We were gone for a weekend and came back to find that the little girl had died postoperatively. I had to deal *with her* that night. This was my first real contact—with my roommate and her relationship with the family and her feelings of this little girl's death. It took quite a while that night letting her really express this.

Other students resisted talking about upsetting experiences, probably because conversation of this nature stimulates feelings which are difficult to manage, and these students preferred to keep themselves under control. Some students were so disturbed that they had hysterics or prolonged bouts of weeping after they left the scene of a traumatic episode. Many reported disturbances in sleeping and eating habits for days, occasionally several weeks, following such experiences.

During the interviews with students it became apparent that those who had not talked about these significant experiences during the crucial first days following the incidents were left with a residue of unresolved reactions, often seriously disturbing ones. Many strong feelings, and sometimes resistance to opening up old wounds, came to the surface when the student was asked to describe her experiences with dying patients. As one student said, "I haven't gotten over it yet." By comparison, students who had access to conversational support following significant and difficult experiences appeared better able to appraise the reality of what had happened, including their own part in it.

There can be little doubt that many encounters with death leave a lasting impression, even though incidents may not consciously be remembered most of the time. It is also quite clear that the psychological effects of these experiences are directly related to the dimensions of familiarity-unfamiliarity with death and adequate-inadequate performance in the presence of death. The ultimate outcome seems to depend on whether or not the student has the opportunity for help and understanding during the critical period immediately following a significant incident.[12] First encounters with death profoundly affect the students as persons. These initial experiences also profoundly affect how they will cope with death when they become practicing nurses. For some students, coping with death is accomplished by choosing a nursing specialty which reduces the chances of contacting death, or by selecting a job which achieves the same ends. The part played by these incidents in the socialization of the nurse has probably not been recognized sufficiently, nor has the lasting effect of traumatic and difficult incidents been fully appreciated. How these encounters with death and with dying patients influence the developing nurse identity is considered in the next chapter.

[12] The *timing* of assistance by others may have crucial significance for subsequent psychological events in the lives of those undergoing significant and crucial experiences. See J. S. Tyhurst, "The Role of Transition States—Including Disasters—in Mental Illness," *Symposium on Preventive and Social Psychiatry*, Walter Reed Army Institute of Research (Washington: U.S. Government Printing Office, 1958), pp. 149–169.

Chapter 6 | Nurse Identity
and Care of
Dying Patients

Experienced hospital nurses have well-developed
sets of expectations about dying patients and the work which
comprises their care in the hospital. These nurses are familiar
with the many different and often difficult work problems associated with dying patients, such as making decisions which can
affect the hastening of death, the handling of negligence evaluation (both individual and collective), the managing of interactions with patients and their families, the administering of the
"nothing-more-to-do" phase of dying.[1] In addition, these nurses
have developed many "out" mechanisms for limiting their own
involvement while in the stressful business of caring for the
dying patient, especially as the end draws near.[2]

[1] When the patient no longer has a chance for recovery either through
natural processes or through medical assistance, he can be considered in the
"nothing-more-to-do" phase. See Barney G. Glaser and Anselm L. Strauss,
Awareness of Dying (Chicago: Aldine, 1965), pp. 177–225.
[2] *Ibid.*, pp. 226–256 discusses the relationship between composure strategies

The nurse student is not aware of these problems initially but discovers them, or parts of them, during the course of her training. While in school the students acquire expectations about dying, and these expectations are used in the development of a nurse identity. Whereas previous chapters dealt with the effects of encounters with dying on the individual student, this chapter is concerned with a more total picture of the student as a young woman in the process of becoming a nurse. The outcomes for basic students in nursing are described first. By way of contrast, a second section considers what the beginning staff nurse learns about dying that may be different from what she learned as a student. A third section describes the identity conflicts experienced by graduate students in nursing through the impact of an educational program which attempts to alter previously established patterns of providing care for dying patients.

Conditions Which Contribute to Identity Stresses

Dying is not the only disturbing problem with which students must deal as they undergo the process of becoming nurses, and there are other situations which provoke feelings of helplessness. Hospital life brings students into contact with crippling and suffering and ways of living markedly different from their own. Students who have been relatively protected from the "realities" of life can be shocked when they are suddenly confronted with events which precipitate sharp emotional reactions.[3] Other situations are disturbing because the events are personally meaningful. The birth of a baby is especially poignant to many because they are anticipating the experience of motherhood for themselves.

---

developed by nurses and the social structure of the hospital wards. See also Jeanne C. Quint, "Awareness of Death and the Nurse's Composure," *Nursing Research*, 15 (Winter, 1966), pp. 49–55.

[3] In "The Socialization of the Student Nurse," *Nursing Research*, 8 (Winter, 1959), p. 22, Thomas Rhys Williams and Margaret M. Williams report drastic emotional reactions to intimate patient care involving six specific aspects thereof: defecation-urination, sex, death, disfigurement, patient and family reactions to pain and death, and odors and handling soiled linens and other materials.

These young women are upset by such matters as viewing a prolonged and difficult labor or the birth of a deformed baby. Ross
made this observation.

> Birth and death, then, are two of life's crucial experiences which
> student nurses cannot avoid and which they encounter more
> realistically than the average girls of their age. They may see
> the more distasteful aspects and the agony that often accom-
> pany them. Moreover, they may have to take part in the drama
> and sense their own inadequacy both in bringing life into the
> world and in preventing its leaving.[4]

It is not just that students in nursing are suddenly exposed to
life in its less pleasant forms. For many the experience takes
place during a crucial period in their lives—the transition from
adolescence to adulthood with its responsibilities and choices,
including the expectation of marriage and family. Discussing the
impact of hospital life on students in a diploma school of nursing, Zinberg and his associates noted,

> We know that nursing educators have puzzled for some time
> about the difficulties faced by adolescent girls entering the world
> of the hospital, as exemplified by the drop-out rate and the high
> ratio of psychiatric referrals when such facilities are available.
> It is our contention that some of this is explained by the recog-
> nition of how much unconscious conflict is stirred up by the
> realities faced in nursing education. These are far different from
> those of the college student, and the extent of the anxiety gen-
> erated in nursing schools calls forth in many girls unusual
> rigidity and dependence on rules. Thus dependence, plus ex-
> cessive expectations from the story-book "men and women in
> white" leads to disillusionment. Too, the patients, by virtue
> of being ill, are permitted emotional reactions of unusual in-
> tensity. The neophyte nurse is faced with the reality of a pro-
> fessional lifetime requiring an appropriate emotional response
> to a remarkably demanding relationship.[5]

[4] Aileen D. Ross, *Becoming a Nurse* (Toronto: Macmillan of Canada, Ltd.,
1961), pp. 245–246.
[5] Norman E. Zinberg, David Shapiro, and Walter Gruen, "Some Vicis-
situdes of Nursing Education," *Nursing Outlook*, 10 (December, 1962), p.
798.

Mauksch found that few eighteen-year-old girls in a hospital school were prepared for the support-seeking and helpless behaviors of sick adults. The school's course content offered few conceptual guides for helping the student understand her own reactions or the dynamics of her interactions with patients. The students resorted relatively rapidly to a "professional behavior"—dignity, defense, distance—to cope with many threatening situations.[6] In describing the identity stresses of students who had two years of college life prior to entering nursing, Davis and Olesen found two sources of conflict in addition to the impact of nursing itself. The students were disconcerted when categorized as nurses rather than attractive young women. They found themselves immersed in a female world—with much of their life centered around getting along with women.[7]

Clearly the process of becoming a nurse involves identity stresses of several kinds, and dying is an especially distressing problem because of the high value attached to recovery by the healing professions. The patient who dies is a reminder of professional failure. There are also difficult decisions and serious interactional problems which nurses confront when they work around dying patients. Because of the characteristics of school assignments, nurse students experience some work problems frequently—such as talking with dying patients; but they have fewer opportunities to encounter other problems—for example, the decision whether to give or withhold a narcotic when its administration might hasten a patient's death. There is no orderly progression of student experience with death and dying, and there are differences in the amount and kinds of experience students have during their basic education as nurses. Each nurse student defines her role in providing care for dying patients on the basis of the expectations

[6] Hans O. Mauksch, "Becoming a Nurse: A Selective View," *The Annals of the American Academy of Political and Social Science*, 346 (March, 1963), pp. 88–98.

[7] Fred Davis and Virginia L. Olesen, "Initiation into a Women's Profession: Identity Problems in the Status Transition of Coed to Student Nurse," *Sociometry*, 26 (March, 1963), pp. 94–96.

that she learns through these somewhat variable experiences. These expectations are incorporated into a developing nurse identity.

The Basic Student in Nursing

The Development of Death Expectations in Nurse Students

Through their assignments to patients, all nurse students develop some expectations about death and dying—including what is considered to be appropriate behavior for the nurse. By listening and watching, the students become aware of dying as a hospital phenomenon which has a variety of possible characteristics. By active participation they engage in certain nurse activities concerned with the care of dying patients, but they do not necessarily participate in *all* the activities of which they become aware. Because of differences in direct experience with death itself, some students develop a rather broad and full set of nurse expectations, whereas others develop fragmented and incomplete notions about dying as hospital work and the specific problems which staff nurses face.

In spite of their variable personal encounters with dying, there are some general learnings which all students pick up sooner or later. They learn that death can be a blessing as well as a tragedy.

> Idealistically, the medical and nursing professions prolong life. And this is what the public's image is. This is what our self-image is. But when you see sickness every day, and you see relatives who are suffering prolonged agony watching a member of their family go downhill, stay downhill. Financially unable to afford care, emotionally drained, you realize that death can be a blessing—not only to the person who is the patient but to those around him that love him.

Out of vicarious as well as direct experience, the students shift from an idealized layman's perspective that medicine can "cure all ills" to a more realistic appraisal of what is involved for physicians and nurses. All students become aware of the "nothing-

more-to-do" phase of dying, and the limits of what can be done
to promote recovery. One girl described her reactions as follows.

> Many times when the doctor has said that this person has just
> so many hours to live, the normal response from a student who
> hasn't been in the hospital for that long a time can be, "How
> cruel he is." Here you are trying to do all you can, and yet
> as you go, you see that there are only so many things that you
> can do for a patient. It isn't as dramatic and life-saving as you
> expect.

Knowledge about dying begins to assume specific dimensions as
the students undergo experiences whereby their general or vague
ideas about dying are subjected to the test of reality. For example,
all students know in the abstract that everyone must die, but
the first death of "my patient" brings to each student the reality
that it does happen. Out of such experiences a student develops
expectations about specific types of patients.

> I prepared him for open-heart surgery. I didn't even check the
> next day. I just assumed he was going to be in ICU, so I went
> up on the weekend to find out when he would be coming up
> from ICU. I thought I'd just go to see him as I felt sort of
> a tie, having prepared him on the last day. It just didn't regis-
> ter really that he had expired on the table, and so when the
> next week my instructor assigned me to an open-heart patient
> who had surgery about the same time but who was recuperating,
> I guess this was when I realized that I was somewhat anxious
> because I was very careful reading the chart. I wanted to know
> everything about this patient—before and how long she had
> been in surgery, very meticulous about finding out these things.

From the death of one patient this student learned to apply some
expectations about dying to a second patient. She sought for
specific cues to assist her in making an appropriate determination about the possibility of dying because "heart surgery" now
carried a new meaning for her.

For nurse students the development of expectations about dying includes two dimensions of learning—the establishment of

expectation types and the reading of cues whereby the different types are recognized.[8] The learning is a complex process whereby general notions become particularized. There are at least three ways by which the process apparently can take place—the student asks for a given experience; learning comes by surprise; understanding emerges slowly out of an accumulation of previous learnings. In the incident just described, learning came about because the student had assumed life, and death came as a surprise.

When students ask for an experience, it is generally with the idea that certain experiences provide the kind of preparation necessary for being a nurse. A student made this comment about herself.

> I asked if I would be allowed to observe the postmortem care. I thought I should get it over with because you have to face it sooner or later, and although I didn't want to take full responsibility for it because personally I don't think I have my organizational things down pat enough, procedurewise and all that. I'm kind of lost in a web of red tape, and get all mixed up. I didn't know just how to react to seeing a dead person and actually working on them. I knew that I would have to do it sometime so I requested that I could help.

Even when students ask for certain experiences, however, they are often surprised by the tangible realities that they encounter. Requested assignments generally bring unexpected additions to the student's repertoire of death expectations. A student who had requested an assignment to a women undergoing chemotherapy for terminal cancer was quite unprepared for the sudden com-

---

[8] Defining a patient as dying depends on two variables—*certainty of death* (the degree to which the defining person is convinced that the patient will die) and *time of death* (the expectation of when death will occur, or of when the question will be resolved). In combination, certainty and time yield four "death expectations": (1) certain death at known time, (2) certain death at unknown time, (3) uncertain death but known time when question will be resolved, and (4) uncertain death and uncertain time when the question will be resolved. See Glaser and Strauss, *op. cit.*, pp. 16–24.

ment, "God, I wish you would let me die." The student described her reaction in this way.

> Sort of a panic. In a way that's not very clear—just thinking what can I say now. She cannot mean it—that was the first thing. Then, what shall I say to see if she does mean it, if she really feels this way.

Although she knew the prognosis was poor, the student did not anticipate such a direct confrontation of the wish to die, nor did she know how to respond to it. The student's expectations of acceptable dying behavior did not include this manifestation. She learned that persons facing death may want to talk about matters for which there are no answers.

Sometimes the determination of a patient's dying status comes about through the slow process of identifying several different cues and using them to redefine the situation, as the following example indicates.

> After he was in about two weeks, the doctors decided to do a peritoneal dialysis. This is when I really started taking care of him. One of the doctors asked me to special him on the PM shift. This man had nephritis, but he was holding up real well, and at the time I did not know this was a chronic condition. I thought this was just a temporary procedure to alleviate his discomfort until his kidneys were functioning again because he was in almost complete renal shutdown. I thought he would pull through. He was just the type that had to, you see.

> The next day I came on, and they had stopped it. I took care of him again. During that night he actually began hallucinating and started becoming very bizarre, and I started to think— my gosh, this is really odd, this just doesn't happen. I was so busy with all the physical aspects of taking care of this patient that this just went through my mind. I tried to keep him as oriented as I could because he was really scaring me—his hallucinations. So I talked to the doctor that night, you know. Before I did, I looked at his medications. He had been on one of the cortisones so I thought with my mediocre mind that maybe it was the effect of the cortisone. So then I went to

the doctor, and he said that he has chronic glomerulonephritis, and this more or less confirmed what I thought.

The next day I went on, and he was progressively worse—in fact, almost nothing. His blood pressure was in the 200's. Then when the doctor said that this was the chronic stages of nephritis, I pushed it out of my mind. I can very vividly see this and recall this. Just pushed it out of my mind and took care of him for the next week. Then his output started to increase and his blood pressure went down, and so I thought—great, they're wrong. So then they started to do another dialysis. About a week later I really realized, you could just tell that this man is not going to pull through.

Through a gradual process the student changed her expectations about the patient's future as the cues available to her began to point in only one direction.

As this incident clearly shows, the development of an expectation type depends on two learnings—knowing the sources for obtaining cues and reading the cues with some degree of accuracy.[9] The inability of the beginning student to make a correct assessment of clearly visible cues is vividly demonstrated in the following comment.

The first death was in my first rotation, and each rotation lasts for six weeks. The woman was quite elderly, about eighty-five. She was a CVA (cerebrovascular accident), and she was semiconscious—responded every once in a while. Her extremities were extremely cold. I tell you this because these are things that stick in my mind. We called her Emily for the sake of calling her something. I didn't realize that she was dying, but I knew that she was. My intellect knew, but my spirit wouldn't realize it until one day I came to work and my instructor told me very calmly, very sweetly, that my patient had gone to heaven. It was rather a shock. It seems funny to say this, but she seemed sweet and kind of resigned to her fate even though she couldn't respond to me in my verbal way

[9] The sources for obtaining cues are many: They include the chart, the seriously ill list, physicians, nurses, teachers, the patient himself, direct observations, reading of related reference materials.

or even smile. But you did feel that she was responding to you every once in a while.

From a student perspective expectations about death have a limited and particular meaning—the student is focused on learning how to recognize dying and how to act like a nurse by doing the right thing and by behaving in a professional manner. Moreover, she defines dying primarily in terms of the final days or weeks of life, and she is given a rather fixed picture of a nurse's responsibilities during that period. One student described what she was taught in this way.

> As far as the patient is concerned, we have to keep him as comfortable as possible and try to alleviate his pain by following the doctor's orders. As far as the family is concerned, we were told that this would be a difficult job. You have to watch what you are saying. If they come up and ask such things as, "What's wrong; is he going to die?" you can't answer but you refer them to the doctor in a tactful way. You have to watch your answers but you have to be personable, and try to answer the questions without involving yourself or committing yourself or the patient.

From their teachers the students obtain generalized ideas about the nurse's responsibility for the dying patient and for his family. Through the patient assignment this responsibility begins to take specific shape, but the reality of what the nurse must do is not anticipated. For instance, the general directive to provide psychological support for the family does not tell the student *how* to proceed when she finds herself faced with a specific problem —the grief-stricken family. A senior student described this incident.

> I think the one I remember the most occurred last summer to a young woman who had cancer. She had a child, a girl about twelve, and her husband was present. This one incident was very outstanding to me. She had a very painful death and it was quite sad for everybody. There was an awful lot of psychological support that was needed by the family.

When I went on duty about 7:00 in the morning, I gave her morning care. The doctor said she would have about an hour and a half to live, that she was very bad. After giving her morning care, the rest of my responsibility was to handle the family. The young girl was crying, and her husband was walking in and out. He was asking various questions, and the doctor had already talked to him and said that she had a very short time to live. All I could do was to give some support and just take things as they came. At one point the little girl became quite hysterical, and I took her down to the coffee shop, and we gave her something to eat. Yet she wanted to be with her mother and it was her mother's wish that she be there. So I just stood by her, and as far as taking care of the patient, it was just seeing that the oxygen was on and checking the vital signs.

I think this hit me emotionally because I just felt so sorry for them since she was such a young mother and the daughter was so young, and I thought that they expressed their emotions so freely, and it just hit me. The picture of the husband and the daughter still remains in my mind.

Through this assignment the student participated in two difficult and unsettling aspects of the last stage of dying—the death watch and family handling.[10] She learned something about composure management of the distraught family, one of the emotionally upsetting problems that hospital nurses often face.

Assignment Conditions and Encounters with Staff Nurse Problems

The management of composure is only one of the difficult problems deriving from staff nurses' work with dying patients. There can be other emotionally distressing problems—difficulty in providing painless comfort; concerns with negligence; personal involvement with patient or family; decisions relative to the hastening or delaying of death, e.g., the use of "nonrescue" tac-

[10] See Glaser and Strauss, op. cit., pp. 226–256 for a description of some common problems faced by staff nurses and the strategies they develop for coping with these emotionally distressing and difficult matters.

tics; interactional strains with patient, family, or with physicians. Nurse students are exposed to bits and pieces of these problems, and their opportunities to learn how to cope with them in a systematic way are often limited.

Although there are some problems all students experience— such as learning how to talk with patients who are not to be told they are dying—other problems are experienced in a less predictable way because assignment conditions either block a student off from the experience or make it available in an attenuated form. For example, most students experience personal discomfort when they are unable to relieve a patient's pain during a one- or two-day assignment. However, fewer students undergo the more difficult experience of trying to provide painless comfort, through a period of several weeks, to a dying patient whose pain becomes progressively worse and almost impossible to control. When a student has the latter experience, it is because the school makes use of prolonged work-type assignments, or because the student has the experience while she is employed outside the school—most commonly during the summer months.

When a student works in the capacity of a special nurse, she can be fully exposed to the difficult problems of providing care to the dying. Under such conditions the student does not have access to the mutually protective strategies used by the ward staff, for instance, the use of rotating assignments so that no single nurse carries the brunt of a difficult patient assignment.[11] The student experiences the full impact of what it means to carry responsibility as a nurse. One student made this observation.

> You have to do what you think is right, and if you feel that, you know, becoming close to somebody you can help them more. Because we did. Three of us girls took care of this pa-

11 Isabel E. P. Menzies in a study of a London hospital concluded that the nursing service developed a particular kind of social system to protect the individual nurses from the anxiety-producing aspects of patient care. See "A Case-Study in the Functioning of Social Systems as a Defense Against Anxiety: A Report of a Study of the Nursing Service of a General Hospital," *Human Relations*, 13 (May, 1960), pp. 95–121.

tient, and three of us became very, very close with him and the wife, and they counted on us quite a bit, you know. After he died, I was glad because it was so much suffering and he was uncomfortable. Then I really started to think about, you know, euthanasia. Not so to speak, but just forgetting all this last-minute emergency stuff that runs into so much money and just prolongs lives so much.

Through this assignment the student encountered some of the most difficult problems and decisions which the hospital nurse faces in her work with dying patients. As a student still in the process of learning, she was extremely vulnerable to the impact of personal involvement. In her words,

The wife had progressively known this was coming, so she finally realized he wasn't going to last too much longer. He finally passed away. I was not there, thank heaven. This is one time where I wouldn't have been able to support the wife or to function as a medical nurse. I'm sure I wouldn't have. If I had been asked to be on duty as a special towards the last, I would have refused because I just get too emotionally involved sometimes, and you still can't function.

As a special nurse for several weeks, the student had a maximum exposure to distress with a minimal amount of protection from personal involvement. This is quite different from the more usual student experience of having a relatively brief patient assignment.

Many students in the baccalaureate program had a very limited exposure to the daily problems that the nurse must face in providing care for dying patients in the hospital. By comparison, students in the other basic programs did encounter many of these problems. In fact, some students had intense experiences with extremely distressing situations, including the problem of providing painless comfort for several weeks. In either case the majority of students had limited opportunities to deal with their own feelings about death or to develop some degree of comfort in working around dying patients and their families.

This is not to say that individual students did not have incidental experiences which enabled them to become comfortable with selected aspects of the dying-patient situation. However, the happenstance rather than planned nature of exposure to these problems encouraged many to avoid dying patients because they did not feel adequate in knowing *what* to do and *how* to do it. As a result, two patterns of avoidance emerged. Some young graduates, particularly those who had very traumatic experiences as students, actively avoided hospital work which might bring them into contact with dying patients. Other young graduates developed what might be called a passive avoidance of contact with dying patients. They cultivated a professional demeanor which protected them most of the time from personal involvement in emotionally distressing situations with patients, and they used this "professional" approach whenever encountering dying patients.

The Development of Professional Demeanor

Out of vicarious as well as direct experience, most students learn to keep themselves emotionally distanced from dying patients. In fact, all students develop a professional demeanor which they employ to a greater or lesser degree to avoid personal involvement with patients in general. One senior described these changes in herself.

> In caring for patients over a period of time and getting to know the family, I had a tendency not to want to get tangled up with the patient or with the family. I did so by not questioning as much as I could. In any relationship you can make it more intimate than it is, or keep it from getting that way. Then rationalize by saying, well I'm helping this person while I'm here. There are little ways you can help without draining yourself so much. I feel that I have changed a lot since the first summer as an aide, which stands out in my memory as being not only a very enjoyable time, but also a time when I got too involved—more involved than you really have time to in one lifetime. When I would go home, on days off, I would think I'd rather be back and see what my patients are doing. I'd come back and be very anxious to find out what had hap-

pened during the interim when I hadn't been there. Now, I've gotten more hard and callous and I try to avoid getting that involved.

For many students the impact of personal involvement comes about through a meaningful experience with a patient who dies. A student who had worked very intensively with a patient prior to cardiac surgery made this observation about herself.

I found out about her death sooner than her doctor. I had gone to ICU to ask how she was doing and was told she had died. My feelings, of course, I had become so involved in this that I was upset about it, and I tried to find the husband but he had already gone. We had become very close, just talking about it. He was really afraid that she was going to die, and he wasn't going to be able to see her again. Thinking back on it now, I know that I really did invest too much of myself, you know, knowing that she did have a chance of dying.

Intense involvement with a patient and family in combination with a death which was not completely anticipated caused this student to consider how to protect herself in future encounters with dying patients.

Actually I have never become this involved with a patient who has died, and I think that if I do it again, I will remember what took place and be more aware of my own feelings. I think that I kind of went in feet first in this. I think I will do a little bit more thinking, although what I do with the patient may turn out to be exactly the same. I think I would be more aware of what I am doing, rather than just going by instinct and empathy.

In a similar way a student can be upset by a death which carries high social loss, as the following incident shows.

I remember one patient in particular. He had leukemia, and this hit me hard. This man came in with a sore throat, and hoarse; a very nice man. He was a divorced man about thirty-two. His ex-wife never came to see him but his children were always allowed to see him, and they were twelve, eight, and six. They were always coming in to see him, and he never left the hospital.

I felt sorry for his children. Every time they came it hurt me because he knew and he was trying to tell them all the time. All he was saying was, like he was trying to crowd it in the last few days, everything he would like them to know. "You study hard now and learn all you can—never stop studying." Always words of wisdom; that was really rough.

He told me once—well, we try to get him to eat and he was so nauseated that—he would say, "What's the use, I know the end is coming." And he would want it to hurry up and he would say the *only* reason he didn't want it to come faster— he was suffering, and this was quite a statement for him to make—he said, "The only reason I don't want it to hurry up and happen is for the children's sake." He wanted to see them grow up. I think that was probably the most difficult for me— he was there so long.

From incidents such as these students learn to define what constitutes a potentially distressing assignment before getting too deeply involved in a situation. Thus many students plan to avoid working in pediatrics because they cannot tolerate their feelings of sadness when they see children dying. A student told this story.

We had a little boy. That was so sad that every time I would walk by I would start crying. It was really sad. It was sad to see some of the other nurses, like say the harder nurses, that would come by and force him to eat food. I felt that he should be able to do what he wants. He was just darling, just precious, I wonder why he was chosen.

Another student, describing a pediatrics ward in one hospital, said, "It is kind of hopeless situation there. It is very depressing to me. I could never work there." The students learn to avoid wards which have especially difficult terminal-care problems.

The students also develop a professional rationale by which they justify certain approaches as appropriate or inappropriate actions for a nurse to take. To do this the student shifts from a lay perspective on certain matters to a nurse perspective. The following incident shows this process developing.

> The husband was there both days before surgery. He wanted to be with her the morning before, and I had tried to intervene with Dr. Smith to see if he would make an exception in this case, to let the family in before surgery. He disagreed with this and said that he didn't want to make a dramatic exit, down the elevator type of thing. He said that it tended to get the patient a little too highly emotionally pitched, and it wouldn't make the anesthesia successful. Then I tried to interpret this to the husband, and he accepted this as being whatever would be best for his wife.
>
> I was kind of upset that this couldn't be, upset with Dr. Smith. But on the other hand, my professional knowledge kind of helped me in that, because I realized that there was a valid reason for not having the family see her. It turned out that she would not have been aware that they were there even if they had been allowed to come, because the sedation level was so high.

In this instance the student moved from identifying with the family to viewing the situation *as a nurse*, and to do so she had to redefine the problem by incorporating new ideas into her initial perspective. Often this process of change takes place in such a subtle way that the student is unaware that it has occurred. For example, controlling conversation with patients can be managed much of the time by the use of techniques which students have already learned as middle-class Americans. The assignment context permits them a wide range of individual decisions with respect to such matters. However, they also find that these behaviors can easily be incorporated into their definition of "being a good nurse."

> They say that to be a good nurse you have to be a good listener and, really, I found that if you just go into the room, some patients are the type that really tell you something about their condition or their problem. Others really withdraw and would rather not talk about it. I think that there are certain ways you

can get a patient to tell you, if you want to. I think that's something that you can try to get out of them, but then, this is my own personal feeling—they would rather not talk about it, unless it is something that should be brought out for medical reasons.

Through direct personal experience lay decisions about how to converse with patients become justified by a professional rationale.

The more I get into nursing, the more I let the patient initiate conversation. I think I was a little too eager at first. I did have a patient with cancer, and they did a biopsy and decided just to give her radiation treatment. Her prognosis was poor. I was with her the morning she found out her prognosis.

I was prepared when I went up that morning, so I did bring it up, but I don't think it was the wisest thing. She talked about death, that she didn't fear it, and she talked about living longer than her brothers and sisters. She was only forty and she felt that there was an afterlife. She also started crying a little bit, and this made me uncomfortable.

I thought about the situation afterward and evaluated it. This is my opinion. I don't think that she was expressing her deep feelings about this. I think she was expressing a sort of objective point of view, and it wasn't a reality to her yet because she didn't feel bad, she felt good—so she was facing it intellectually rather than emotionally. I think that it was too premature, I think that when the time is right a patient will give his view.

Many students learn to let the patient decide whether or not to talk about his illness. This conversational approach becomes justified as "best for the patient." Through an accumulation of these experiences the student builds a professional demeanor which she can rationalize in terms of "patient needs." At the same time, the demeanor serves to protect her from emotionally distressing situations.

Negligence Evaluation and the Care of Dying Patients

Just as a student develops a set of interactional tactics in accord with her evolving nurse identity, so does she also develop ideas about what constitutes good practice in other aspects of nursing where dying patients are concerned. Feelings of negligence can be associated with the following areas: recovery care, activities related to saving lives; comfort care during the nothing-more-to-do phase; or simply failure to meet certain human needs. Through specific assignments students learn to apply general ideas they have been taught, and to build confidence in their abilities to cope with particular problems, e.g., carrying out certain procedures which are important components of comfort care. One student described a meaningful assignment.

> The one patient I remember most clearly was the one I had for two weeks straight. He was a cardiac patient that came in after suffering a stroke. The first five or six days he was fine; he wasn't considered to be dying—only he might have a little paralysis. Then around the seventh day he suffered another stroke and was moved to a private room and given oxygen. He had to be suctioned and his position changed and all. I wasn't there when he actually died.
>
> I got a lot out of knowing a patient like that. It was when I was working in the summertime, and I enjoyed taking care of him and trying to help him. It was good to be there—little things like turning him so he wouldn't get bed sores and things like that. Because you read about this but you don't really understand it until you are confronted by it.

This student was faced with a responsibility about which she was uncertain, and she had a chance to see herself functioning successfully as a nurse. During the first days of such an assignment, a student's concerns about being evaluated as negligent—that is, unable to provide good patient care—show in her comments about herself. As another student said in describing her conversation with an instructor, "We talked about my being slow in getting started. I felt that this bothered me because I thought that this was a detriment to my being a nurse." Through direct participation in patient care, the nurse identity begins to take form. The students refine their ideas of what constitutes negligent nurse performance. They evaluate themselves as negligent or non-negligent by comparing their own behaviors against these emerging standards. They develop an image of themselves as nurses, capable or incapable of providing good nursing care. When a student has assignments which permit her to see herself performing successfully in providing care to dying patients, she begins to develop a picture of herself as a competent nurse. If she does not have the chance to practice these activities, she has no way of assessing her abilities to perform them competently. Her image of herself as a nurse has an area of uncertainty.

When the opportunity to practice leads to negligent outcomes, the student tends to visualize herself as incompetent. Incidents of the latter sort have a significant influence on the developing nurse identity *when* the nurse responsibility imposed by the assignment is beyond the student's capacity, and she either makes a mistake or is unable to meet the assignment requirements to her own satisfaction. A student described the impact of such an experience.

> I was on for two weeks taking care of four patients who were not seriously ill. They were ambulating and near discharge. Then I was assigned to care for this woman who was forty-eight. She had a teen-age son and a husband who came to visit her. When I began caring for her, she was precomatose. She had cancer, and it had presently spread to the brain. The first morning was bad, and then the second morning that I went in—we were working full mornings at this point, the doctor's orders were to give terminal care, and I didn't seem to be able to function at all that morning, even enough to give her a decent bed bath or to turn her as often as was ordered. She had labored breathing. She was catheterized, had a rectal tube, and oxygen and IVs. This whole thing about keeping a patient alive when you really feel there is no hope. It's terminal care, and you have all these intravenous feedings and oxygen to keep her going. To me it just seemed that dying in itself was enough

for the family, and then to be put into a situation to care for her when I had never taken care of a seriously ill patient. I didn't feel that I got any support from my instructor, more of it was constructive criticism—or not so constructive—as to where I couldn't function and I had better think about this and look into that. I needed someone to tell me this. I needed someone to talk to me and to let me get my feelings out. I had nightmares while I took care of her, and I couldn't function effectively. It was just too much.

In describing her reactions to this assignment and its effect on her, the student made these comments.

I felt a great deal of responsibility toward the family and toward her, and I felt inadequate to do any of them. I don't think I have gotten over that experience yet. I dread that ward, and I don't like to go near it. If I had been assigned there again, I think that I would have done everything in my power to get a change—probably without telling people why because I feel that I'm expected to have different feelings about death by now. I feel that it would be detrimental to my standing in the school if I admitted these feelings. It was one bad experience.

The development of a sense of adequacy as a nurse can be blemished by a single traumatic episode in which negligence evaluation plays a critical part. Often the young graduate chooses her first work position either to gain experience she did not obtain as a student or to avoid situations which left painful memories. Encounters with death critically influence these decisions.

The Beginning Staff Nurse

First-Time Experiences with Death

Young graduates come to their first jobs in hospitals with variable amounts of experience in providing care to dying patients. Some have had a great deal of experience and others have had very little. One thing they have in common—they are now part of the hospital staff, not outsiders to it. For nurses who had limited chances to encounter death or dying as students, the first job often provides important first-time experiences. One girl witnessed her first death and described it in the following way.

> The doctors had said she could go any time, and they didn't know, or she might last. I went into the room and took the pulse. It was real slow, and all of a sudden it speeded up and you couldn't count it. I was just amazed. I had never seen anything like it before. So I thought I'd take a blood pressure more or less. The doctor had just taken it, but I thought I would too, just to see if I could get it, and I did. Then the practical nurse who is over fifty-five—she's been in the game for a long time—said, "Let me take it, too, just for practice to see if I can hear it." Just as she finished taking it off, all of a sudden there was this gasp. I looked at her and her eyes rolled back, and that was it.

> At that time I was just so grateful I had the practical nurse with me because she had seen a lot of this and it helped. The first reaction was to get the doctor so I stayed in the room, although I really didn't know what I could do. I felt it would be better to stay with her. The doctor came right in and tried to massage her, and she gasped a couple of times, and he quit. I thought of my own feelings at the time. I thought I was doing real well. It was what you might call a model death. Although my knees were shaking, I wasn't afraid. My knees were shaking from tenseness. It wasn't at all frightening, and I was surprised, being the first actual death I had witnessed.

Her words convey a student's viewpoint—amazement upon viewing the unexpected, taking advantage of the chance to practice, relief that she was not alone, and gratification that she performed well in a new and tense situation.

Another young graduate had her first emergency experience when a patient developed cardiac arrest during the change of shifts. As team leader she found herself running around getting supplies for those gathered around the patient, and relaying messages among the doctors and nurses directly involved in the event. She talked about the experience thus.

Then I went back to the room and asked if I could do anything, and nobody said anything, so I thought what should I do now. Should I go and get the other people ready for the daily routine, and then let these people handle the situation—which seemed logical to me. Besides that, I think I really used that as an excuse because I really didn't want to be in there. So I gave report—and all the time I was giving the report, I was just shaking. Then I went back to the room, and she was still not breathing on her own. But everyone had a job, so I left. After that I started with the day. Of course, it was very unnerving. I had a very confused morning as a result of that one thing that happened. I imagine my reaction would have been different if I was right in the room, participating in it.

It was a very frightening experience. I used to know this person, and these things affect me. I wasn't thinking straight, and everything seemed to go wrong. Everything seemed to happen at once—and just trying to think of everything that was supposed to be done and trying to be clear in my mind. But I don't think I really felt it, the experience, like being in there with the patient. This was my first time. Nothing like this happened in training.

Her description carries a mood of uncertainty and tension. It reflects the disorganizing effect of a new, and very important, work encounter experienced by one who is meeting it for the first time. It also conveys an implicit, as yet unanswered, question about her own ability to recognize an emergency and to implement life-saving activities should they be needed.

The Realities of Hospital Work

Experiences like the two just described are expected in the sense that they are recognized as traditional nurse activities, but there are other experiences which also take place. All beginning nurses must now learn to cope with the practical problems of work associated with particular wards. As staff members, they must deal directly with situations which, as students, they often did not have to face, e.g., the problem of deciding how to cope with a difficult family of a dying patient. Learning how to cope with families under emotionally distressing conditions is an activity for which few guidelines are available. One young nurse described the following incidents.

We had a little two-and-a-half pound premie that had died. It was just pitiful. It was a baby of an unwed mother, but she wanted to keep the baby. It was having blood trouble because she was RH negative. It died in the middle of a transfusion. It was so pitiful because it was so tiny, and it was the orangiest color from the blood. I had to wrap it up and put it out in the anteroom. The family wanted to come to see it, so I had to show it to them. This was quite stressful. The body of the baby itself didn't bother me so much, but showing it to the family.

The mother, plus her boyfriend, and her parents and a sister. A couple of them came right in and looked at it closely, and they just stood there and watched. They didn't say anything; there wasn't a sound. The father wouldn't—he stood out in the hall—they tried to get him to come in but he wouldn't. Well, I figured that the best thing I could do was to just stay there and let them look as long as they wanted to, and not say anything, and I did. I think it worked out pretty well. It's an awful trying situation and hard though, because you really don't know what to do or how to be best support to the family.

As is often the case each nurse decides for herself what is "best" for handling these unanticipated problems. Other difficulties, however, may precipitate collective problem solving by the nursing staff. A new graduate on a cancer ward described the staff's response to one difficult patient.

He is very demanding. He wants ice chips and then he wants cold water. You bring it to him and no, he doesn't want it that cold, he wants it a little bit warmer. Then it's too warm, and he has us constantly going on. We find ourselves, over and over again, probably three or four times a day, in little informal sessions having our small team conferences; discussing, you know, what's going on with John now. At times you lose your temper with him, and other times you don't because basically everyone kind of understands that John is dying in the way that he lives, which is pretty appropriate.

She was learning to participate in collective *ad hoc* decision making, a ward strategy which tends to appear when the staff as a whole face an emotionally difficult piece of work.

The young graduate's first job may bring her face-to-face with difficult choices she had not anticipated—for example, the decision to use rescue tactics to save the patient's life when she would prefer to let him die, because he is suffering. The doctor may leave loose sedation orders to ensure painless comfort until the end, but it is the nurses who decide how often the drug will be given, and the young graduates may be unaccustomed to this practice.[12] Those who choose to work in large urban hospitals may well be surprised and unnerved by the changing character of life-death decisions, and the new responsibilities that nurses are expected to carry, such as the use of external cardiac massage for cardiac arrest. They can also be upset by the unexpected consequences associated with new and uncertain medical therapies—for example, the terrible shock which follows when a young patient with a renal transplant pulls the shunt apparatus out of his arm and bleeds to death. The young graduate can easily blame herself for failing to recognize the patient's suicidal intent because she was so preoccupied in learning about the unfamiliar technical procedures.

A problem faced by many new nurses is that of amalgamating an ideal about nursing with the reality of hospital work. One girl described her internal conflict of interests.

One was a dying patient, and another was a patient handling her own feelings about her husband who had died and trying to help her with that. These both happened on the same day, and I was also assigned to six other patients. All of the eight involved a lot of physical care and treatments and all this kind of stuff. Since I was just starting out, I had lots of feelings about doing my work well. But still I had lots of feelings about giving emotional support to these two people, and yet there were pressures of getting the work assignment done. So I talked to the head nurse about it, whether or not this was just some-

[12] For a more complete description of certain of these problems, see Glaser and Strauss, *op. cit.*, pp. 204–225.

thing that I would have to learn how to deal with—get my work done quickly. You hear this old school business about assessing priorities, yet I think when the supervisor comes around at ten in the morning, if your beds are not made and your baths are not done, you are rated as a poor to middling nurse. I don't think anyone wants to work in a situation where you are considered to be that.

As might any new employee, she turned to her co-workers for advice. She had this to say about the results.

I am convinced that I am not going to get into a system where I am going to feel bound to get everybody's bath done by ten. I feel that it is far more important just to stop and give an hour or two to these patients who are really crying for help. I can't give it a lot of times but at least you can stop. Some of the nurses suggest, I have talked to a couple of them, and they said that a lot of times you can be doing things like changing their beds and also listen to them. Well, maybe that is so, and maybe I will be able to do that, but right now I just don't think that is right to do. I don't know whether this is because I am just not able to do both things at the same time, but basically I feel it is not morally right to do because it is almost as if you are saying—okay, I will listen to you but just move over and let me do my work and get out of here.

She was facing the task of incorporating what she believed was good nursing within the framework of a given ward system— and not without difficulty. The work routines and staff expectations interfered with her aspirations for providing unique and personalized care as needed—in this case, being available to patients who wanted to talk about dying, at the time when the patients indicated a readiness to talk.[13]

[13] Corwin found that graduates of degree programs experienced more role conflict than did diploma graduates in their efforts to function within the hospital work world. See Ronald Corwin, "The Professional Employee: A Study of Conflict in Nursing Roles," *American Journal of Sociology*, 66 (1961), pp. 604–615; also Ronald G. Corwin and Marvin J. Taves, "Some Concomitants of Bureaucratic and Professional Conceptions of the Nurse Role," *Nursing Research*, 11 (Fall, 1962), pp. 223–227.

Difficulty in communicating with physicians was frequently described by young nurses who had been taught that patients have the right to a reasonable explanation of what is happening to them. A young graduate who took her first job in a community hospital run by physicians in private practice found herself constantly in hot water with either the head nurse or with one of the doctors for talking "too much" with patients. She could not explain her actions satisfactorily to these authorities. On one occasion, telling a patient the name of a diagnostic test precipitated a ward crisis. No longer protected by her student status, this nurse was learning that what she believed was good nursing practice could bring her into open conflict with those in authority.

Through the restrictions and expectations imposed by others in her work world, the new graduate redefines her responsibilities to and her relationships with patients, including those who are dying. In a similar way the graduate nurse who returns to school for advanced education may unexpectedly find herself put into new relationships with dying patients by virtue of her teacher's restrictions and expectations.

The Graduate Student in Nursing

The Impact of Assignments to Dying Patients

The nurse students who returned to school for advanced education came with well-established ways of behaving as nurses. As part of graduate courses in medical and surgical nursing, some instructors used a teaching focus which caused some of the students to reexamine their ideas of the nurse role in providing direct care to dying patients. In their efforts to help students develop a more personalized approach to nursing practice, the teachers used an assignment strategy which precipitated tremendous personal involvement for the students. These teachers used a familiar assignment situation—nurse with patient—but with a different emphasis and different expectations. The teachers emphasized the interactional parts of nursing care, and they expected the students to report back on what they were doing during their interactions with patients. The old nurse behaviors were no longer readily available to these students. Many found themselves facing role conflicts in terms of self, patient, family members, teachers, physicians, and other nurses.[14]

These role conflicts came about because the students were expected to behave in ways which did not agree with the nurse behaviors they had already established through previous training and work experiences. The old nurse defenses were no longer available. Assigned to patients with chronic diseases, the students were encouraged to stay with a single patient throughout his hospitalization. Consequently, the nurse, again a student, became involved with the patient in a personal way. If he died during the assignment, his death became an intensely meaningful experience for her. Frequently the patient's death brought a self-evaluation of negligence, with feelings of guilt, helplessness, and loss of power. One girl made this observation.

> The week before he died he sort of began to talk more about his feelings. But I think he was mostly bewildered. He never realized that he would die this soon, and I wasn't with him the last week. In fact I made a point not to be there because I had a feeling he would die, which made me feel even more guilty about being out of the situation when he was able to relate to me in a way that he wasn't able to relate with the other nurses. So he never really got near to death as a subject again, and I think he very much would have had I let him go on, but I would change the conversation to books and flowers and anything I could think of at the time.

Many students encountered difficulties when their patients wanted to talk about the when and how of their dying. Prior educational experiences in nursing had not prepared the students to cope with this type of conversation, yet the assignment purpose

[14] Not all students accepted the teacher's approach, and some successfully evaded involvement. These differences are probably related to their variable backgrounds—educational, experiential, personal—and to their different educational motivations—reasons for returning to school.

made it difficult for them to run away. As a result, conflict followed.

> He was only given three or four weeks at the longest. He was extremely frightened and was always asking to talk about his feelings. I couldn't let him. I even recorded what I was saying, and this sort of thing, and became very depressed for two weeks because I became involved in it myself. Every time he brought up feelings I would change the subject. If he mentioned the word *death*, I would practically walk right out of the room without giving him any warning.

> When I was with him my feelings were mostly that I wanted to get out of the situation. I understood him but I wanted to get out of there. That was all I could think of. Then I felt so guilty about this until I began to talk to the other nurses on the ward who said they felt the same way. They couldn't stay in the room very long, and I realized that I was extremely sympathetic toward him, and that I was closely identified with him.

Not only did these assignments cause difficult and distressing problems, they also precipitated memories of past encounters with death—often traumatic ones. One student recalled this incident.

> What really bothered me was one who died suddenly. I was supervising a house at night and had nothing but students on the floor, and we were very busy. She had a convulsion and seizure. We called the doctor who was a neurosurgeon. At that time neurosurgery was relatively new at that hospital. There were some differences of opinion as to what she had—there was no definite diagnosis. After the surgery, we gave demerol. Suddenly the picture changed remarkably—the pupils fixed and very comatose. I didn't get any satisfaction from the intern, and she died all of a sudden in spite of everything we could do. Calling everybody, and I remember the doctor being very upset—why didn't we call him. It was a conglomeration of many factors, and I blamed myself for the fact that this woman had died. And *that* I remember quite vividly. I was very upset about that. The administrator was shocked, and she went to the autopsy and came back with the report saying what had

happened. It proved that I *didn't*, but that morning I felt that I had done something wrong.

Considerable time in class was given to reviewing and reliving stories from the past. New encounters with dying patients provoked many thoughts about previous encounters with death, particularly those in which personal negligence or unexpected shock had been critical factors. The seminar often became a ventilating session in which the students shared their painful memories and provided emotional support for each other.

Some Problems Encountered in Changing the Nurse Role

These assignments brought the students into new kinds of relationships with patients and with family members. The teachers encouraged them to interact openly with the patients and to intercede with their families. When they undertook these tasks, the students often found themselves in new and tension-producing circumstances. A student who had been working closely with a cancer patient described the following experience.

We got her actually involved in solving her pain problem, how she was going to manage at home, and we got a VNA referral. The doctor seemed to take a little more active part in it, and the staff, too, in supporting her. Then I got there the next day, the patient was to be discharged in two days, and she had had a myocardial infarction and was in ICU. I went to see her, but it was then time for class. She didn't respond too much, and I kept missing the family. I had to chase up and down the floors trying to find them. I left a message with the supervisor to call me if anything happens. After class, I went back upstairs. I got back twenty minutes after she had died, and I was kind of appalled in a way.

I was frustrated. I felt during those three hours that maybe I could have been helpful to this patient. I didn't know whether I could or not, but it is a possibility. I felt more frustrated about the family than I did about the patient. I only met the husband once before, and he seemed kind of nervous around her. It was all of a sudden a complete reversal of plans, and

I didn't know where to go from there. I thought the best thing I could do was to make myself available to the family, they were pretty upset. The doctor laid the facts on the line with them. The husband just sat there. I sat down beside him, and he moved away from me as soon as he could. Considering what had happened, he didn't even cry and he looked at me real funny. The younger son, I thought this was a very difficult time for him, he looked me right in the eye. I got the feeling of being nailed to the wall. Then the elevator came and he left. It was upsetting. It seemed to me that the family was never really brought into the situation.

The students were encouraged to work closely with the family but often were frustrated either because the opportunities for direct contact were limited or sporadic, or because they did not know what to do when they did make contact. When they tried to compensate for these problems by asking the regular nursing staff to help, they were often frustrated by a lack of interest or by direct avoidance. One student described the student position thus.

It is so different when you work with a staff. You get to know everybody, and then you can do things together, and you can suggest ideas and maybe you can suggest them to somebody who has a little initiative, and they'll tackle it, and no one is threatened by it. I have established a relationship with one nurse and so far, I can say anything that I want to her, and she agrees with me and will try what I suggest, and I'll try to use her suggestions. But she herself isn't able to communicate with the rest of the staff because, I mean, they don't seem to have much communication between them. Even when one suggests something, the others drop it off flat. It just never seems to work out.

From the viewpoint of the staff, the students were outsiders. They were also trying to implement new nursing practices. Because of these two factors, both threatening to the staff, the students were likely to encounter resistance when trying to enlist cooperation from the regular nursing staff.

The students also found themselves in new relationships with their teachers and with fellow students. The characteristics of the patient assignment led to intense personal involvement with previously avoided patient problems, but the students were also expected to talk about this involvement in class. The teachers were making them responsible for what they said and did during interactions with patients and families, and the students found themselves faced with feelings of helplessness and anger. One student complained about the lack of direction from teachers.

> I would like a few views to fight with, or at least to have some kind of interchange rather than a purely listening relationship. I feel that an instructor who has had some experience should be able to give me better clues.

Later in the year she described herself as functioning in a completely different way with patients, and she now referred to the same teacher much differently.

> She didn't force me in any way. She told me I could pull out at any time I wanted, and I knew she would be receptive to any action I took. However, I don't know that anyone else would have been able to give me the support I needed because I was changing my whole view of life at the same time. I had a whole new orientation as to how to deal with other people.

> I *did feel* such a failure and my instructor was willing to point out little things that were positive because my level of expectations for myself is so much higher than I am able to achieve that I had to bring it down a little bit.

For this student the turning point came when she was able to permit a man who had recovered from cardiac arrest to talk about death.

> He was able to mention the words *death* and *dying*, and I was able to repeat for him the word *death* throughout the conversation, so he began to look at it as a realistic possibility in the near future. Then he changed from his discussion of death to discussion of his finances, and what really concerned him about dying was that he would leave his wife alone. It was only a half-hour interval of working out a solution of finances

and realizing he had it pretty well set. In the end he was no longer hostile, and the whole ward the next day seemed to be saying to me that the patient has lost so much of his hostility toward the disease. This was an extreme reward to me.

Often the teachers provided support through individual conferences, but class discussions were also helpful to many students. The latter derived additional support through being able to talk about their problems with other students. One student described the value of a particular class.

It seems extremely threatening, yet I can hardly wait to get to class. It's anxiety provoking. I find myself giggling at the darndest things and they really aren't funny, but I'm releasing tension. The one thing that seems to be coming clear is that I block in talking about cancer.

I feel a little more secure talking about it. I know cancer is a loaded subject for me, and I ignored the fact for a long time. This morning a patient brought up the subject, and I'm not ignoring it like I was.

In this class we can focus on it. If I want to be shook up, I can. It's okay to be shook up in this class, and every one of us is working on the same thing so it's a kind of mutual support society. I want to learn to face cancer, dying, whatever it is, and this is to me the best way to practice and get the support either from the teacher or from each other, and we try.

Many of these students were learning new ways of communicating with dying patients and their families. To do so they had to revise their notions about being a nurse. One student summarized her ideas.

I think a lot of things have helped a lot. Realizing that the patient wants to feel in control, and he has a sense of dignity that he feels must be maintained; that he has to be able to break down in an accepting atmosphere so that he doesn't have to lose control in front of people where it matters to him. This is a very real role of the nurse. To let the patient break down when he can, in an accepting atmosphere, and also in helping relatives; to be able to accept this as a need and not to judge, but to help them through it in whatever way they can.

The process of change was not easy, and teachers and students alike found themselves having to face and to deal with their own feelings of helplessness. One of the teachers made this comment.

This kind of involvement is not familiar to these girls. The group this year has gotten into this early because of the diseases they were treating. They suddenly realized they were not making these people well. They said, "We've always thought of it as getting them out of the hospital, and you've done a good job, pat yourself on the back." They were aware right away that this was different, not like they had done a good job, but that these patients were not going to get well. So they were beginning to think of death in a different kind of sense—not as specific incidents but as the ultimate end of patients that they were taking care of. And this was very upsetting to them.

Rewards, Gratification, and the Nurse Identity

Nurses get their professional rewards and satisfactions principally from participating in activities associated with the preservation of life. Many nurses get little personal satisfaction from their interactions with dying patients, because these assignments provoke helpless feelings. In addition, nurses have had few specific guidelines for knowing what to do when faced with several recurring problems which arise in interaction with the dying—the patient who wants to talk about his forthcoming death, the patient who cannot tolerate being left alone, the patient whose behavior expresses strong anger or intense fear.

For nurses who work in the hospital, especially in a general hospital, still other aspects of assignments to dying patients are troublesome and distressing. The nursing staff carries major responsibility for providing care when recovery is no longer possible. During this period nurses often must make decisions which conflict with their notions of their primary occupational purpose—

to help patients recover.[15] Often, too, the provision of comfort, whether this be physical or psychological, is not easy to achieve. The inability to offer comfort during the final days of a patient's life adds to the nurse's feelings of helplessness and frustration.

Becoming a nurse is not an easy process, and the student encounters many identity stresses during her educational experiences. In coming to terms with some of these stresses, she internalizes a nurse image which gains gratification primarily from assignments in which she helps the patient get well. Among the students participating in this study the majority had limited opportunities to learn how to achieve satisfaction from assignments to dying patients: they developed a nurse identity primarily committed to recovery care.

There were a few students who learned to communicate openly with dying patients and their families. Some were graduate nurse students who revised their established identities as nurses by learning how to get rewards from relatively open interaction with dying patients. The others were undergraduate students in the baccalaureate program, where the teaching emphasis on psychological care of patients had a profound effect on the student's developing nurse identity. However, only a few of the undergraduate students learned to communicate openly with dying patients and their families.

The undergraduate student who developed this ability followed a somewhat atypical pattern in her student career. Characteristically, she encouraged patients to talk and to express their feelings and met no major conversational setbacks during her first year in school. The student did not live in the dorm or with her nurse classmates during that first year, thus she had limited access

[15] The doctor can add to the nurses' problems by transferring a high proportion of responsibility to them. Conversely, the doctor can make the task easier by sharing responsibility and by supporting the nursing staff when serious decisions are required. But the dying patient is also a difficult work problem for physicians, and they too have received little preparation for coping with the personal reactions accompanying this serious professional problem. See August M. Kasper, "The Doctor and Death," in Herman Feifel, ed., The Meaning of Death (New York: McGraw-Hill, 1959), pp. 259–270.

to informal class advice on how to avoid getting personally involved in difficult patient situations. In a sense the influence of student culture was peripheral rather than central as far as her personal development was concerned. She worked in a hospital during the summer months and had her first encounter with death under relatively easy circumstances. Her student career was marked not by sporadic and unrelated encounters with dying patients, but by a clustering of emotionally meaningful experiences. Usually these experiences involved several different dying situations, with one serving as a significant turning point.

Characteristically also, each of these students had a significant person to whom she turned for advice and support when she encountered these tension producing experiences—and this person was readily available whenever the student needed to talk. One turned to a chaplain whenever she needed help in deciding which decisions to make.

> First of all I called him to come up to talk with her because I felt that even though I was ready to verbalize, I didn't feel that I could offer her as much guidance and direct help as the chaplain. We had worked together before. So I called and asked him to come up. He did. Actually she told him exactly the same things—her fears of dying. I told him what I was doing so he would know what we were trying to do. He was with the husband when she died, and he helped him quite a bit. The husband had asked for me, he wanted to talk to me, but the chaplain didn't know where I was. I felt badly that I couldn't see the husband afterward because I had worked a great deal with him, and with the chaplain. I went down to his office and talked quite a while afterward.

Another student gave most of the credit for her ability to relate with dying patients to a nurse teacher who had supported her through a difficult assignment to a man with cancer. She looked on this assignment as *the* crucial experience in her development as a nurse. In her words, "I learned that you cannot force another person to accept death, but you have to work with them in terms of where they are and what they can do." At a later time on the pediatrics ward this student was able to work with a youngster who had leukemia rather than to "fall apart" like her classmates. She said of herself, "I was upset inside, but I was able to be more objective." She also stated that she could not have developed this ability without having gone through a significant, emotionally distressing, personal experience with a dying patient. Just as the graduate students who revised their identities as nurses, this student had to experience deep feelings of helplessness in a supporting atmosphere before she could learn to relate openly with patients who were facing death.

In Summary

The process of becoming a nurse involves identity stresses of many kinds. Providing care for the dying is especially stressful because of the high values attached to recovery care by the nursing and hospital cultures. These values are further reinforced by the expectations of the public who hold in esteem the life-saving abilities of doctors and nurses. Because basic educational programs in nursing do not systematically assign students to dying patients, the students have these experiences under a wide variety of circumstances. As a result there are great differences in what the students learn about the care of dying patients as a form of hospital work. Despite these variations their identities as nurses providing care for the dying include the development of a professional demeanor useful for avoiding emotional involvement with these patients. Each student's image of herself as a capable nurse is greatly influenced by assignments in which negligence is a critical factor. Traumatic experiences can produce a nurse who carries a deep sense of personal inadequacy.

Encounters with death also contribute to the developing identity of the staff nurse, especially during her first job in the hospital. The beginning nurse may have her first experiences with death at this time. Also important, experiences with dying patients bring the young nurse face to face with the realities of her work world. She learns to modify her role to conform with the restrictions and expectations imposed by it, as does the nurse who returns to college for advanced education. Because of the teacher's requirements that she alter established ways of interacting with dying patients, the graduate student in nursing is likely to experience role conflicts which are both threatening and upsetting.

Among the students interviewed, some graduate students learned how to interact relatively openly with dying patients, as did a few undergraduate students in the baccalaureate program. The latter followed a somewhat atypical career pattern, including limited exposure to the effects of student culture. In both instances the students developed this ability by directly facing their feelings of helplessness in caring for dying patients. The next chapter considers how these students—and the others—contributed to the lives of patients who were dying.

Chapter 7 | Some Consequences
for Dying Patients

Sometimes nursing students contribute in very meaningful ways to the lives of patients who are dying. Sometimes they contribute very little. This chapter considers what happens to the individual who is living through the final period of his life, or is living with the possibility of imminent death, and in the process is brought into contact with one or more nurse students. The following analysis was based principally on indirect evidence—obtained through interviews with nurse students, with their teachers, and with others involved in providing care for these patients. To a lesser extent some data were procured directly through conversations with dying patients themselves. In consequence, the chapter describes an incomplete and somewhat limited picture of what happens to these patients as a result of their encounters with nurse students.

What is likely to happen to dying patients when they are used as assignments for students essentially depends on two conditions.

The different assignment contexts in which patients are used as school assignments contribute to a variety of possible consequences, some of which are described in this chapter. In addition, a student's prior experience significantly influences what she is *able* to do in a given assignment and what she *chooses* to do. Either purposefully or unknowingly, students can behave in ways which lead to critical experiences, negative or positive, for the patients to whom they are assigned. What the student does, of course, is affected by the assignment context in which she and the patient meet. Among the many characteristics which define the assignment context, the length of an assignment is especially influential in these matters.

The Influence of Assignment Length

When school assignments are made for only one or two days, the dying patient ordinarily can have little more than superficial relationships with the students who are assigned to provide care for him. When a series of students are assigned to him for short periods of time, he constantly must adjust to a new nurse. These assignment practices may add to the dying patient's problem of establishing human contact with any one person and may effectively increase his isolation from meaningful interactions during this crucial period of his life.

By comparison, the lengthy assignment to a student may provide the dying patient with compensations for some of the more impersonal aspects of hospital living. In a positive sense, the prolonged assignment can be meaningful to the dying patient simply because he does not have to interact with new nurses every day. There can be compensations in the form of physical comfort measures provided by one person who is familiar and takes account of his likes and dislikes. The student may also provide human companionship that the dying patient is unable to get either from his family or from the hospital staff. The student may not always know what to say, but she can provide human comfort in ways other than by conversation. One student described this experience.

I find it hard to say something to him about his death because I don't know if he wants to or not. He seems rather despondent about it. He worries about his wife a lot—what she will do afterward. But I found that talking isn't the only thing that I can do. He seems to greatly appreciate small favors such as washing his face when he's been perspiring, and other things of this nature. At one point I walked in and he took my hand and just held my hand. This was all. He didn't want to talk, and I realized the only thing for me to do was just to stand there and stay as long as he wanted someone in the room. It seemed to me that he was alone and didn't want to be alone, so I figured the best thing for me to do was to stay with him. The last two days I have not been assigned to him, but I go in as frequently as possible just to say, "How are you doing? Is there anything you need?" He seems to appreciate this. I still find myself thinking, "Is there something I can do for this man, some other little thing that might make things a little easier for him?" But I especially noticed that he didn't want to be left alone.

Sometimes the student brings meaning into the dying patient's life by engaging in conversation which brings him back into the realm of the living. Another student made these comments about a young man dying of leukemia.

When I took care of him at first, he was kind of irritated. He didn't like people. Well, I just stayed with him, and we got to talking about certain things. We just happened to have a few things in common. I think he realized I wasn't a dope, and we got to talking about things I had said, where I had been. I had traveled, and he had traveled. That was one of our common meeting grounds. So we had a good relationship. I took care of him about two weeks, and we spent half our times debating and discussing things. He enjoyed this, and he didn't have too much family here.

Not all students respond to prolonged contact with the dying patient in a positive way. Some students react to the lengthy assignment by depersonalizing the patient. They provide physical care in a routinized manner and withdraw from active interaction, thereby effectively blocking the patient's efforts to establish human contact. Some students may even abandon the patient by asking for a change of assignment. These practices are not unique to students, however, but are also used by many graduate nurses and other hospital employees when they are assigned to dying patients. Analysis of the data shows that the student who has had few if any prior assignments to dying patients is more likely to provide human comfort during a lengthy assignment than is the student who has had prior assignments of this nature. The student who has already experienced prolonged or difficult contacts with dying patients is prone to keep herself detached from this kind of personal involvement during subsequent assignments to those who are dying.

Whether the assignment is short or long, what the student chooses to do is influenced by her prior experience. Many student actions during assignments to dying patients are governed by what the students learn through experience with other nurses, both in the classroom and on the hospital wards. Students also make many decisions on the basis of what they are expected to do as nurses, and on what they are expected to report back either to their teachers or to the ward nurses. What happens to dying patients is significantly influenced by the fact that the students do not have to account for many of their actions.

The Unreported Events in Patient Assignments

In her encounters with dying patients the student can do many things which she does not have to report to anyone. For example, she is seldom held accountable for what she says to patients. Her actions can cause conversational successes as well as conversational blunders as far as the dying patient is concerned, but the student may or may not discuss these events with her teachers or with the hospital staff. In fact, the student may even be unaware of the effect of her actions on the dying patient.

In many instances, particularly when short assignments are used, students and patients move past each other with relatively little meaningful interaction occurring between them. Consequently, there are numerous conversations which result in relatively neutral outcomes for dying patients. There are some occasions during these short assignments when students perform meaningful functions simply because they happen to be present during periods of crisis. For example, a student becomes a listener because a dying patient has desperate needs to talk at that point in time. Although she may not always recognize the value of her actions, a student who does not withdraw from this kind of crucial encounter may provide the patient with a much wanted opportunity to talk about what has happened. Thus a man who has been told that he has inoperable cancer wants to talk about what this announcement means for him and for his family.

> When I walk into the rooms it is dark because, you know, they are usually asleep. I heard a noise. It startled me, and I looked in the bed and there was nobody in the bed. He was sitting in the chair. He and I got to talking and his doctor had told him that he had cancer, that day. He had been in a couple of weeks before. He was taking it pretty hard.

> He was just sitting there, so I switched off the light. He didn't have a roommate that night. I had said, "What are you doing there?" He said, "I'm thinking." So I thought—well, there is something wrong. I couldn't quite remember what was wrong with him. So I switched off the light. It was quite late at night so I had time and sat there and talked to him for awhile, and just let him talk.

In describing what they discussed, the student commented,

> Primarily the house and his family, but a lot of it was material goods at first. You know, something was material. And then it was more, "Why does it have to happen to me, I have lived a decent life. I haven't done anything wrong, or gypped anyone or anything." He was just throwing out questions, and I didn't get the feeling that he was expecting any answers.

This man reminisced at great length about his work, his family, his retirement plans. The student defined his situation thus.

> He went on and on, and it seemed like he was trying to face it. It was just too much for him to handle at that time because the staff nurse went down there, and he talked to her some. We talked it over, and we both came up with the same ideas. He needed someone to talk to.

Another patient facing death may want to cry because she is upset and afraid, and the student provides her the opportunity by staying in the room—even though the student herself may be upset by the experience, uncertain about what she is doing and anxious to leave the room.

A student can also retreat when a dying patient makes this type of conversational overture, or she can effectively block him from talking or weeping. A striking observation is that very frequently the beginning, inexperienced nurse student in her spontaneous and human interactions with dying patients is more apt to make a positive contribution to the psychological well-being of the patients than is the more experienced nurse (or senior student), who is inclined to respond in a well-conditioned, institutionalized manner. In a sense, the young and inexperienced student has not yet learned to use the profession as a shield to protect her from an open encounter with the dying patient and his feelings.

A student's actions can produce conversational blunders too, and the inexperienced student is a likely candidate for initiating such results. Sometimes a student unwittingly contributes to a patient's knowledge of what is going on—again because she happens to be present when a crucial incident occurs. The inexperienced student is most likely to give away the truth when a patient unexpectedly asks, "Am I going to die?" In response to the surprise question, a student may blurt out "Yes," or she may burst into tears and leave the room. A teacher reported the following incident.

> I'm thinking of one in particular, of a student who was talking to a patient who has a possible malignancy. Something came out in the process report. She asked the patient if he was feeling any stronger, because he had been weaker. He said, "No." She realized that he was always looking very jovial, and suddenly she opened her mouth and said something like, "But

you are trying to kid everybody?" I don't think she realized what she was really saying. He said, "Yes, I try to fool people, but I can't always do it. In fact, I'm not so sure I fool myself." And then she said, "What kind of work do you do?"

This is a first-year student, and I'm sure she has no idea that she turned him off and jumped to another subject, because I don't think she meant to get involved in that.

The student may also react to a patient's direct question with a commonly used nursing practice of saying nothing, which may also be interpreted as an affirming sign by the dying person. Direct disclosure to a patient of his forthcoming death is a "goof" according to usual nursing standards, but it may have a very positive effect on the patient who has suspected his future and wants to know about it. Inadvertent disclosure may be upsetting to another patient because he was not expecting the news or because he now wonders whether he can trust his doctor or his family. Because these conversations are often not reported, neither the hospital staff nor the teacher may know about them unless the incident causes the patient to become unduly disturbed. In this event the incident may lead to a generalized ruckus, with an upset nursing staff and an angry physician—especially if the physician did not want the patient to know.

During their first encounters with dying patients, students are most likely to make interactional blunders in much the same spontaneous way that they sometimes contribute warmth and human understanding. Lacking familiarity with the situation (and often not knowing that the patient is dying), the inexperienced student can innocently ask a question which causes the patient to burst into tears, or to become angry. If she does know that the patient is dying, she is likely to wonder how she will respond if he wants to talk about his dying. Under this kind of tension, she may well answer the suspicious patient's unexpected inquiry as much by the look on her face as by what she says or does. Quite unintentionally a student can confuse a patient by encouraging him to open up, then cut him short when he starts to talk about matters which cause her to feel uncomfortable. What looks like a blunder to the student may not necessarily be bad from the patient's perspective. On the other hand, there are times when actions of this sort simply add to the dying patient's psychological burden and personal distress.

In her encounters with dying patients and their families, the student also meets situations in which she must knowingly decide whether to give out specific information about the patient's condition or his future. As is true with nurses in general, students make many such decisions on an *ad hoc* basis—depending on how they think the patient or his family will respond and on the perceived requirements of the specific situation. Thus a student may decide to tell one patient about another patient's death, even though this practice is generally discouraged by nurses and physicians. One student described her conversation with a former cancer patient.

> One day he came back. He had been coming back to the clinic and then visiting Mr. S. who had a private room. He came back the morning after Mr. S. had died, and I had just come back and found out. He came up to me (we had talked quite a bit every time he came in) and said, "What happened to my young fellow?" I stopped and thought, "Should I or should I not tell him?" What are the rules on the floor? I had never bothered finding out. What does he know—I can't tell him. Then I thought, "You don't want to tell him because you're so upset." Finally I decided, knowing him. He was accepting his disease better than almost anyone on the floor. Also I don't think he would have asked the question, knowing the state Mr. S. was in, unless he had an idea.
>
> So I just said, "He died." I was careful not to say he passed away because I noticed all the nurses say that, and it bothers me. It's being afraid to say what actually happened. He just looked at me and said, "Oh, he was *so* young and it was *so* hard for him." I said, "Yes." We sort of shared. I think both of us were close to tears for him and, you know, I felt better after that. I think he did too.

In this instance the imparting of information led to a warm and meaningful experience for the two persons involved.

Undoubtedly students give out a great deal of miscellaneous

information in their conversations with dying patients, often with little effect on subsequent events. They can also transmit information which is incorrect or misleading, not uncommonly because they are uninformed about particular facts. For example, one student told a patient and his family that they could visit him on the morning of his surgery, only to learn afterward that the surgeon in question would not allow this kind of activity. The student then faced the problem of changing their expectations by interpreting the doctor's policy to them.

Quite unintentionally a student may contribute to a patient's confusion about what is happening to him because the "facts" she gives are at variance with the facts given by the physician. She may continue to tell him that he is "well," although the physician may have let him know that his condition is deteriorating. She can also give misleading information to a patient or a family because she misjudges the situation; for instance, a student's estimate of a patient's time of death can be inaccurate, thus resulting in the family not being present when the death occurs. The imparting of misleading or erroneous information is not unique to students. However, students (particularly in the beginning) are likely to be less well informed about many aspects of dying than are the regular ward nurses. Inexperienced students also have not yet learned to be cautious in giving out information which can easily backfire because of its unpredictable nature.

Although students may choose not to report many events which take place, they are certainly held accountable for many of their actions. In fact, they are sometimes responsible to more than one authority for the same patient assignment. The assignment condition of reporting to multiple authorities affects what happens to dying patients because of what happens to students when they are accountable for their actions to more than one person.

Nurse Responsibility and Accountable Assignments

When working relationships between the teacher and the ward nurses are cooperative, the chances are decreased that a dying patient will suffer because a student gets caught between two nurse authorities. When cooperation exists, the assignment environment tends to be supportive for the students who can easily turn to the staff when they encounter difficult patient problems. When assistance is readily available, the student is likely to make use of it with better results for the patients. For example, she feels free to ask for assistance in moving a dying patient who has considerable pain instead of attempting this activity by herself and thereby precipitating additional discomfort for him.

If, in addition to being cooperative, the teacher and ward staff are consistent in their views about what constitutes nursing practice, the student's actions are likely to be consistent with those used by the staff. This may mean, of course, that a student learns to avoid or to depersonalize dying patients because these are the views which predominate on the wards. On the other hand, if it is expected that the nurse takes time with the dying patient to provide physical comfort and simply to be with him, then this is what the student is likely to do. Students put into practice those activities that they see being performed by other nurses and that are approved by them. When a student works side by side with a nurse who is comfortable with dying patients and sure of herself in providing comforting care, then the dying patient benefits both physically and psychologically. The evidence suggests that students, in cooperation with other nurses, offer the most effective care to dying patients when the patient and his family are open and accepting of his forthcoming death.

When working relationships between teacher and ward staff are strained, patients as well as students can suffer the consequences. For example, if the staff members withhold information from the student and the teacher, the student can say or do the wrong thing with a dying patient because she doesn't know enough not to do so. On wards where this kind of tension exists, students may not feel free to ask for help. Dying patients can suffer physical or emotional consequences of many kinds when the students and ward staff do not exchange information and work cooperatively together.

Sometimes ward tensions are high because the teacher and the staff have divergent views about nursing practice. Even though their teachers may encourage the students to behave in certain ways, the students usually conform to the ward nurse's standards, partly, if not completely, in order to get along with the staff and to complete the assignment. When students are caught between two sets of standards, they move toward the practicing nurses' viewpoint because these are the nurses they see in action. Also their teachers are not always there, and the students are then directly accountable to the staff. Not uncommonly, students are criticized, sometimes quite unkindly, for their actions. They learn that certain behaviors are not considered acceptable by the staff, and they begin to modify their ways of relating with patients. Under strained work conditions, the ward staff may also react by assigning the student to the "difficult" patients. Such actions can have a snowballing effect on the student who, in turn, reacts by "taking it out" on the patient, with less than adequate physical care being one possible result.

The assignment practice previously described also has some long-term effects. Its punitive nature reinforces a tendency, already present in many students, to stereotype certain patients as "difficult." As is also true with medical students, nurse students define patients as "good" or "not good" on the basis of student values.[1] In general, preferred patients are those who recover, provide "good learning experience," and are cooperative with the student. Within the student culture dying patients are not considered preferred patient assignments. This suggests that an interaction between student culture and nursing culture encourages the development of negative attitudes toward dying patients. The practice of negative stereotyping can lead to less than positive outcomes for many patients. For example, one woman who was

[1] In one study of senior medical students, twenty-three out of a sample of twenty-seven preferred patients with acute illness to those with chronic illness. The latter were "said to be more demanding, more difficult to work with, more uncertain of themselves, more dependent and passive, more depressed and hopeless." Robert S. Ort, et al., "Expectation and Experience in the Reactions of Medical Students to Patients with Chronic Illness," *Journal of Medical Education,* 40 (September, 1965), p. 844.

suffering intense pain (associated with bone metastases) described great difficulty in getting relief for her pain because it took such a long time for someone to answer her call light. In discussing her predicament this patient cried and then said, "In all the time you know me, you have never heard me complain. I have always said that this hospital was a fine place, and I felt this up to now. Now it is like a mad house." Because every movement caused her excruciating pain, she did not like to get into a chair. Caught up in the agony of pain which was not controlled by medication, this woman could not move rapidly or easily, and she often groaned loudly whenever the effort was made. In describing her situation, she said, "You lie here, and you think, 'Oh, God, I cannot do that.' The nurses are so clumsy, and you wonder what they are doing." Both she and her daughter tried to talk with various nurses but had no success. The nursing staff avoided them as much as possible. A student described this patient as "spoiled," and stated that the daughter got in the way and made it impossible to carry out such therapeutic techniques as placing the patient in a chair. In this instance negative stereotyping caused additional discomfort for the patient rather than relief for her pain.

It is worth noting that students who were somewhat peripheral in their exposure to student culture were likely to try innovative interactions with dying patients and, by implication, showed fewer tendencies to stereotype these patients. A similar tendency was observed in the graduate and undergraduate students who went through the difficult emotional experience of directly facing their own feelings of helplessness and hopelessness in providing care for dying patients. Also, the latter students did not avoid open interactions with dying patients but instead tried to offer support and guidance to these patients and their families. Some dying patients profited from these efforts; others did not—usually because the students were not always clear about what they were doing.

From their experiences on the hospital wards many students also learned to use the doctor's commanding position in a stereotyped way. Very often they responded to patients' direct questions with, "You'll have to ask your doctor," making little effort to clarify the patients' underlying concerns. This maneuver often prevented these patients from getting much wanted information, and discouraged them from asking other nurses for help. Usually the students did not report the patients' questions to the ward nurses or to the doctors, and the patients' concerns and fears went unnoticed. A few students—particularly those who became psychologically sensitive—sometimes contacted the doctor directly for the patient or took pains to see that a message got to him. One student, for example, was assigned to a man with a pacemaker at the time when he was about to leave the hospital. In talking with him, she became aware that he was very frightened about going home because he would be alone there. He was afraid that something would happen to the pacemaker—that it would stop working, and he would die alone and unattended. The student asked him to write his questions on a piece of paper so that she could give them to the doctor. She then attached the paper, addressed to the surgeon, to the patient's chart. That evening the physician had a long chat with the patient. On the following day this man was a "different person" because he now knew what he could and could not do when he returned home. The student's action had a major effect on his outlook about the future.

As students are exposed to hospital life and nursing culture, they learn to make use of resources highly valued by practicing nurses and nurse teachers in caring for dying patients. One favored procedure is referral to the clergy.

The Use of the Clergy as a Resource

From the beginning, students are taught that the clergy "should be" used as a resource for dying patients. The students also learn that referral to a minister can serve to take pressure off the nursing staff.

> Most of the things that the nurses have said to me are just a few comments about, well, isn't that too bad, or we'll talk about

maybe how the family is taking it, because they're "our concern now." They're all eager to call in the clergyman as soon as possible to talk to the family when they are disturbed about something.

Actual referrals by the students come about in various ways. Some take place because the patient indicates that he wants this kind of help.

I walked in the room, and we were talking. He told me that he had cancer. The doctor had told him, and he would like to see a priest and yet he didn't know if he should. Finally I just listened to him. Then I went out and told the head nurse who called the priest. He came up, and after that the patient was a lot calmer.

Other referrals occur because the student decides that the patient's problem is more than she can handle by herself, for example, a patient who talks about committing suicide.

This man was dying of cancer, and it was terminal. He had a large family, three young boys all under twelve. He was quite a young man himself. He was going through a horrible session of vomiting all of the time. He would sit there and was miserable. He was having quite a bit of pain and was not being handled by the drugs he was getting.

One day I was in there, and he started talking to me about committing suicide. He said that he just couldn't stand it any longer and that he knew that he was going to die, and why prolong it. He said that he thought about it quite a bit and that he had a gun at home. He thought that he could get it and could just take care of himself. He thought about other things, sleeping pills. He told me he started saving pills—I imagine they were sleeping sedations. At this time I just didn't know what to say to him. I could sympathize with him, and I could agree with what he was going through. On the other hand, I felt that this was morally wrong, and that it wasn't my place to condemn his thoughts. As it was, I just tried to let him talk. I felt incapable of giving him any positive support since I was so torn in my own.

I knew that he wanted to talk about it and felt comfortable enough with me to talk about it. At this point I was in my "call the chaplain" stage, so I asked the patient if he would talk to the chaplain. He said that the chaplain had been in to talk to him a couple of times and that he liked him very well. So I asked him if he would like to talk over this problem with the chaplain, and then I put in a call for him. He went in to talk to the patient, and then I told him (the chaplain) what the patient had told me.

Shortly thereafter the patient died, though the student herself was not present. She talked with the chaplain afterward to learn what had happened.

The patient just deteriorated, you know. I think he gave up. He didn't eat. He refused to eat and he died. He just gave up. The chaplain came up every day and talked with him. The chaplain said he really was ready to die and knew that he couldn't get better. The chaplain said that he stopped talking about committing suicide and said that it would be better to meet God just on natural terms than to give up that way.

Sometimes a student indirectly makes a referral to the clergy because something in the situation is disturbing to her, and she turns to the chaplain for personal counseling for herself. On one occasion, a student was very upset because a husband had decided that his wife was not to be told she was dying of cancer. He did not want her to know the diagnosis, nor that the prognosis was poor. Very concerned, the student talked about this matter with the hospital chaplain who began to drop by the woman's room each day. On their third meeting, the woman told him, "You know, I know what I have—that I have cancer, and that I am going to die." The chaplain continued to visit her regularly, and she talked openly with him about her dying, though she continued to pretend with her husband until the end.

As other nurses sometimes do, a student can also make a mistake and can assume that a minister is wanted by a dying patient. The unexpected arrival of the chaplain can be upsetting and discomforting for the patient who does not want or ask for this kind of counseling. A man who had just been told by his physician of the need for a serious abdominal operation thought "my time is up" when the chaplain walked into the room shortly afterward. Whenever a student makes a religious referral without consulting the patient or knowing his wishes on the matter, the chances are that the chaplain's visit may not necessarily be viewed by the patient as comforting and helpful or even desirable. It may instead bring fear or anger or distrust of those who are taking care of him.

One student reported that conferences with the chaplain provided her with help in deciding what to do when she faced particularly difficult decisions during assignments to dying patients. For the most part, these decisions had to do with what to say to the patients when they asked disturbing questions. In experimenting with different ways of providing psychological care for patients, this student—and others like her—were sometimes helpful to dying patients and sometimes not.

Some Results of the Teachers' Psychiatric Emphasis

When their teachers emphasized the importance of psychological nursing care, the students tried out different ways of talking with patients. In their efforts to do what they thought their teachers expected, new students tried to encourage their patients to "express their feelings" or to talk about their problems. However, the students were not always very skilled in talking with patients, nor were they sure of what they were doing. The "rules for providing emotional support" were less clear-cut than the rules governing technical procedures. Consequently, the boundaries between ordinary middle-class conversation and therapeutic discussion of matters not included in ordinary conversation were not clear in the students' minds. Even more confusing and unclear was the problem of determining whether or not one's conversation with a patient was psychologically beneficial for him. Each student resorted to trial and error—with variable consequences for the patients—in the process of developing a conversational approach which was acceptable to her. A student who became a patient for an extended period of time refused to serve as an assignment for other students. She had this to say about being a patient,

> You really don't basically want it to be a nonreflective conversation. This gets pretty dull, and it especially gets pretty dull if you are a nurse. You don't want to get it anyway—you know—as a nurse being a patient. You really would like to have fun conversations, and the aides were the ones who were more fun.

Sometimes the patients had very positive experiences as a concomitant of the student's experimenting. A patient might have a good listener at a time when he wanted to talk, or be able to get information that he wanted, or be able to get a message to the doctor with the student acting as intermediary. In a less positive way, some patients were forced to try to talk when they did not feel like talking. Others were encouraged to open up about their troubles only to find that the students never reappeared. Frequently patients who tried to talk about dying found the conversation quite suddenly and abruptly cut short.

Some students never became comfortable in talking openly with dying patients. Others did not agree with the psychological focus —thus did not encourage patients to "ventilate." However, many students exposed to this viewpoint were inclined to *stay with* patients, even though they themselves did not have much to say. Sometimes a student simply held the patient's hand and listened. Sometimes a student provided an outlet for the family who needed to grieve. One student talked about an assignment to a young girl.

> She was hospitalized in the terminal stages of her illness. What bothered me most was that she wanted to die, and she told me that she did. She knew that she was going to die, and she wanted to. The evening that she died, she was calling out to God to let her die, and her mother just went over in a corner and broke down. I felt that I was giving moral support to the mother at this time.

Although the student was not able to be supportive of the patient in this situation, she was able to give the mother an opportunity to express her grief.

When dying patients were used as assignments for students who were being held accountable for their conversations, the patients often experienced benefits in the form of continuity of contact with one nurse—sometimes counterbalancing an isolation imposed by his family and the regular nursing staff. However, the patients also were subject to liabilities in that the students sometimes asked upsetting questions or left them abruptly when the situation became tense. The patient might try to talk about his forthcoming death only to have the student change the subject. Finally he would stop trying. In many ways the positive outcomes resulting from these assignments countered the less positive outcomes because the students made it possible for the patients to experience support (often unrecognized by the students themselves) in dealing with their human problems—for instance, making difficult decisions.

There are times when a dying patient has been given specific information, usually by the physician, and wants to talk about the significance of the information for his future or for the future of his family. He is often expected to make a critical decision on the basis of what he has been told. For example, a terminal cancer patient who has been given the option of taking an experimental drug with "no guarantee of cure" can use the nurse as a sounding board to help him decide whether or not to take the drug. Although a student cannot readily measure her effectiveness as a helping person in this context, she serves a useful function by letting the patient openly discuss the pros and cons involved in making his decision. In a similar way, a student can be a sounding board when a dying patient has family problems causing him concern.

> She was in her early sixties and had cancer of the liver. She was extremely jaundiced and very weak. Her husband came at 11:00 A.M. every day and stayed until 8:30 at night, and she was so tired. Every time I walked in, there she was talking to

her husband, and smiling as though she didn't have a care in the world. Finally I was bathing her, and we talked about this a bit. She mentioned that her husband was a golfer. He had gone today. Because of her illness, he couldn't get out to the range. Then she said, "I almost wish he went all the time." Then she said, "How terrible I am." And she really felt guilty. Look what she said.

She talked about this—what his coming meant to her. She was finally able to say that when he comes, "He is so nervous and feels so sorry for me that he doesn't know what to do. He sits there and says, 'Can you eat any more? How come you haven't eaten that lunch?' I can't eat a thing. He makes me feel worse so I try forcing some in. Then I feel so sick and there he sits feeling sorry for me, looking straight ahead, not knowing what to say. I'm trying to be cheerful and I can't take it. I *just* cannot take it. I don't know what to do."

We talked about how normal this was, and that it wasn't something that was her *horrible* thought or invention, and she was fine. I asked her, "I wonder what would happen if you were ever to tell him that you thought it might be good for him to do something in the morning, and that you needed the rest because this was making you very tired." She said, "Oh, I couldn't do that."

I came the next day, and she said, "Oh, I wanted to tell you that my husband came. I finally had done some thinking that that wasn't such a bad idea after all. Today he is playing golf, and he is going to every morning. You know, I think it will make the world of difference with him, and also I can be a human being again."

In this instance the student brought relief to a tense situation by listening and by responding in such a way that the patient made a meaningful decision for herself and for her husband.

Often dying patients are conversationally isolated from their families, usually because the family is very upset by the patient's forthcoming death. The patient may be terribly afraid, as was one young woman dying of leukemia. One day she was able to express her fears to a student.

I don't know who brought it up but I am pretty willing to believe that she did, because I don't think I was ready to say, "Okay, I'm ready to hear." She talked about dying. So here we were, two twenty-one-year-olds, talking about death, about her death. What our feelings were and what she has left unfinished. What she was afraid this was doing to her family. Mainly she talked about being afraid. The way she brought up the fear was she was afraid to talk because of what this did to other people—what it did was chase them away. I, having been one of them, could understand that. She couldn't talk about it with her mother because her mother couldn't tolerate it at all.

Sharing such a moment can be a poignant experience for both the patient and the student. It is not easy to let another person express his fears about dying because such talk tends to trigger one's own fears about death. When the student participates in this kind of communion with the dying patient, she makes a significant human contribution during what is for many patients a very lonely period of time.

Some dying patients feel abandoned by everyone unless someone provides them with human contact. These patients frequently behave either apathetically or antagonistically in response to the abandonment. One student was assigned to a twelve-year-old boy who was very hostile and uncooperative. On one occasion he was extremely antagonistic and told her that she was a "bad nurse" because she made him do things he did not want to do. On the following day, however, he apologized, and said that he knew he was taking out a lot on her. "I wouldn't want to make you cry, like I do my mother," he said. Following this interchange, the boy began to depend on the student and to ask her to do the very things which formerly he had refused. One day he asked her how long she would be around that day. When she answered, he said that he had wanted to know because "I like you."

Shortly thereafter, the boy requested that his father stay with him that night because "I like my father and I want to be with him." Neither the son nor the father talked about what transpired during that night, but the student talked with the father before he left that morning for work. According to her report, the father's conversation was rambling with considerable focus on his family and on the tragic situation. Before leaving he told the student that it had been good to talk because he had no one else with whom to talk. He saw himself as having to be strong because his wife was taking the loss so hard.

This assignment was far from easy for the student. The family had decided that the boy was not to be told what was happening. The student talked about what a "rotten set-up" this kind of assignment was. You were told *what not to say* but you were *not* told *what to say,* so that the patient got inconsistent rather than consistent responses from the staff. In addition, there was a tendency for the nursing staff to stay away from patients like him, and sometimes the physical care which they received suffered as a result. In spite of the difficulties which the assignment posed for her personally, the student brought this dying boy warm human contact. She also helped him to attain physical comfort during their brief periods together.

It was impossible for students to give comforting and effective physical care when the assignment expectations were beyond their capabilities. In the incident just described, the student was sufficiently experienced in performing nursing procedures to be able to provide physical care with ease and sureness, thereby assuring comfort for the patient. Some dying patients were not so fortunate.

Additional Effects of Inexperience

When students are new and inexperienced in performing the technical tasks required by their assignments, they are likely to be frightened and unsure of themselves. Serving as an assignment to an inexperienced student can be upsetting and irritating, and far from comforting, to the dying patient who wants to be left alone or who is very tired or upset. Such an experience can add further to the tension of a patient who is already very frightened or who needs the support provided by a nurse behaving in an assured manner. There is also the opposite situation, when patients find enjoyment in "directing" the efforts of the new nurse.

The student is least effective in providing physical care when the assignment is overwhelming in its requirements. Not only is she likely to add to the patient's physical discomfort, but she may not recognize significant changes in the patient's physical condition. She may even make mistakes by improper use of equipment, thus causing further discomfort for the patient or even injury to him. The student is most likely to provide inadequate physical care when she carries this responsibility alone and has little direct guidance and emotional support. The overwhelming assignment can also have far-reaching effects in that the student may develop such an intense preoccupation with avoiding mistakes that she performs technical nursing tasks in a ritualized manner; thus future patients can also suffer the consequences of the assignment. In a similar way, some students develop stereotyped approaches to performing specific procedures—such as postmortem body care— because of the frightening circumstances under which they first are assigned the task. Any overwhelming assignment, especially one which occurs early in the student's experience, has far-reaching effects on her attitudes and behavior toward dying patients.

Students are sometimes given assignments in which they carry responsibility for many patients, although they have had little prior experience in this kind of patient care. When inexperienced students are assigned to be in charge of a ward, they can easily make serious mistakes—even perhaps contribute to a patient's death— because they have little background against which to make judgments about their actions. Moreover, they are likely to be easily panicked by a sudden emergency and may blame themselves if a patient dies.[2] Under these conditions they may also make mis-

2 Mary Burton, Benita Cowlishaw, Helen Hewitt, Thelma Osmond, Sister Mary Bernice, and Kayoko Yoshitake, "Curriculum Development as Applied to the Preparation of the Nursing Student for Her First Experience with the Death of a Patient" (unpublished paper prepared for a graduate course in Curriculum Development in 1960 at the University of Washington School of Nursing, Seattle). On p. 5 note, "In one instance reported in the inter-

takes which they do not recognize, though these actions may not necessarily be harmful to the patients. Perhaps the most far-reaching effects are begun when the student is also punished, either by the teacher or by the hospital staff, for making a mistake. Students who have had such experiences can easily become nurses who are so overly concerned with performing well technically that they see little else when they are assigned to dying patients.

Whenever a student has an assignment which includes a high component of nurse responsibility combined with little prior experience and minimal guidance or direction, the chances are high that a dying patient will receive care which is less than adequate (perhaps even dangerous) by accepted nursing standards. In contrast, when the student has had some experience and encounters a dying patient assignment under conditions that provide her with help and direction, the chance that a dying patient will receive less than adequate care is greatly diminished. He may even receive better than adequate care under the latter circumstances.

A Proviso

There is much to be learned about what *really* matters to dying patients. Much that has been written about death and dying has had a psychological orientation, emphasizing two areas—attitudes toward death and the mourning process.[3] There has been a general tendency to assume that the dying patient's behavior is somewhat fixed and predetermined by his attitude toward death. Some recent publications, however, have addressed themselves to the dying patient's behavior as a function of his interactions with significant persons around him. It has been suggested that the dying patient's acceptance or denial (nonacceptance) of death is

---

views, a diploma program nursing student, responsible for a thirty bed general surgery unit on the evening shift, felt that she had hastened a patient's death by her ignorance of the signs and symptoms of hemorrhage. This was her first experience with the death of a patient and she had been in the nursing program only about six months when it occurred."

[3] See Parts 2 and 3 in Robert Fulton, ed., *Death and Identity* (New York: Wiley, 1965), pp. 79–329.

related to the manner in which he is told his future and to the actions of hospital staff subsequent to the announcement.[4]

Those who have engaged in counseling with the dying suggest that, contrary to the beliefs of many, the approach of death seems to give the patient added psychological strength if he and the therapist enter into an active encounter, the goal being to help him live each moment as it comes.[5] In both publications cited, the authors indicate their beliefs that patients can profit from knowing that they are dying.

Saunders has found that a carefully planned regime for relief of pain, combined with a positive approach toward each patient, provides a climate in which patients dying of cancer feel safe and better able to face the end with courage and with dignity.[6] In hospitals devoted to recovery care, however, the unhurried and personalized approach described by Dr. Saunders is seldom observed. In fact, the opposite tendency is more likely to occur since both physicians and nurses limit their contacts with those who are dying unless medical treatment or hospital routine require their presence. The general practice of not talking to the dying patient about his dying serves to isolate him from meaningful interactions with the significant persons in his life and prevents him from preparing for his own death. If he is surrounded by a conspiracy of silence, then all relationships become superficial. Under these conditions he is also likely to be given physical care in a routinized and impersonal manner.

In the course of learning to be nurses, students sometimes make very positive contributions to the comfort and well-being of dying patients. Under other circumstances, they contribute in less positive ways, often unknowingly and unwittingly. Many of the incidents described by students indicate that the actions of nurses,

[4] See Barney G. Glaser and Anselm L. Strauss, *Awareness of Dying* (Chicago: Aldine, 1965), pp. 119–135 for a discussion of the effects of direct disclosure of terminality.

[5] Margaretta K. Bowers, et al., *Counseling the Dying* (New York: Thomas Nelson, 1964), pp. 74–96.

[6] Cicely Saunders, "The Last Stages of Life," *American Journal of Nursing*, 65 (March, 1965), pp. 70–75.

as well as the timing of these actions, play a significant part in the lives of dying persons, sometimes positively and sometimes negatively. The actual results, however, can only be conjectured until the problems of dying patients have been subjected to systematic investigation as social phenomena within the context of the hospital. Yet it is safe to say that the current system of nursing education neither encourages rational terminal care nor leads to a reflective scrutiny of the specific care that students give to dying patients. Current educational practices have not generally prepared nurses to cope with a very serious and difficult nursing problem. The final chapter considers some ways by which changes in both nursing practices and educational practices might be brought into being.

Chapter 8 | Implications for Change

While collecting and analyzing the data on which this book is based, the author began to speculate about the relationship between what is expected of nurses when they work with dying patients in hospitals and their educational experiences as students. Increasingly, it appeared that nursing students are not being prepared to assume responsibility for many of the complex and serious problems nurses meet in practice. Furthermore, there is every indication that nurses who work in hospitals will encounter more, rather than fewer, problems in which death or dying is a significant feature. According to these findings, the educational approach to the problem of dying patients has been more haphazard than systematic, and the results are something less than what might be desired in the on-going practice of nursing. However, when one views the findings as cultural phenomena— reflecting societal values and beliefs about death—they are readily understandable.

In considering the revision of educational and nursing practices, it becomes apparent that changes are required at several levels. At one level, the changes are pragmatic and easy to identify; for instance, the reported consequences for students indicate the need for systematic planning for assignments to dying patients, especially during the first year in school. At another level, changes are neither simple nor easy to initiate because at issue are basic and deep-seated societal values.

This chapter begins with a discussion of some key issues—points at which the underlying cultural and subcultural values and beliefs strongly affect what is put into practice in nursing and in teaching about nursing. There are three key issues—life saving as a primary occupational goal, the idealization of individual responsibility for patients, and conversation as a component of nursing practice. It will then be relatively easy to consider some specific ways by which these practices might be altered, so as to better prepare nurses to meet the specific problems they will face in providing care for dying patients. Some proposals for change are then considered under the following headings: the first year in school, the use of patients as school assignments, identity stress —the emotional impact of dying, the level of teacher preparation, and the need for counteracting the retreat from hospital work. Finally, the implications of these proposals are discussed as they pertain to the more general problem of the educational preparation of nurses for *all* the stress-producing problems that they encounter as practitioners.

Cultural Values and Nursing Practices

Life Saving as a Primary Occupational Value

As Americans the students bring to these experiences already established attitudes in which death is essentially denied. Direct encounters with those who are dying bring them face to face with the realities of death and precipitate thoughts and feelings that are disturbing. The tendency to withdraw from these situations, which are personally threatening, is supported by the value system within nursing. That is, the high value accorded to life-saving activities reinforces the societal value of avoiding the reality of death. At present both the hospital culture and the teaching practices of many nurse instructors support the primacy of recovery goals, without concomitant direction for attaining the distinctly different goals of helping people to live while dying.

That nurses are "well trained" to think in recovery terms is indicated by an incident which occurred during a statewide meeting of nursing students. A nurse who was conducting a workshop on "Death and the Nurse" asked the students what they would do if they had a terminal cancer patient who suddenly developed cardiac arrest. After much discussion the students decided that they would start cardiac massage, letting the doctor decide whether or not to continue when he arrived. Thus the students made a choice supporting the primary occupational value of saving lives. Yet the decision was required in a context in which life-saving actions might temporarily delay death, but could not ultimately ensure recovery.

The incident clearly illustrates an important facet of nursing life. Nurses make many decisions that directly affect what happens to other people's lives. Nurses also encounter many problems in which the decisions to be made are not of a simple "yes" or "no" variety, nor are the consequences always readily predictable. The nurse's decision to withhold a pain medication may be just as significant in a patient's life as her decision to give it. Her decision to call—or not to call—the physician can have a real bearing on a specific patient's future.[1] Whenever the question of euthanasia is introduced to a group of nurses, the usual response is that "no one has the right to make this decision about another person's life." Yet nurses make many decisions greatly affecting other

[1] So also can the nurse's decision to listen or not to listen to patients and their families have serious consequences. See Nathan Hershey, "When No One Listened," *American Journal of Nursing*, 66 (March, 1966), pp. 532–533.

people's lives. The tendency to think of life-death decisions only in terms of euthanasia is to run away from the occupational "facts of life."

The high value accorded to life-saving practices by the nursing and hospital cultures has caused nurses to develop a limited conceptualization of decision making and nursing practice. Educational programs in nursing have heavily emphasized the nurse's responsibilities for saving lives without concomitant attention to the many other issues involved in actions taken for prolonging life, as well as actions taken for not prolonging life. Nursing curricula have focused relatively little attention on the moral, ethical, and legal considerations underlying medical and nursing practice, especially the patient's rights to be informed when his own life is at stake.[2] In practice, nurses face many problems in which the dying patient's rights are very much at stake, and nurses make decisions that confirm or negate these rights. There are no simple answers to many of these nursing problems, but they exist. Present educational programs have not helped the students to understand the nature of many decisions that nursing work requires or to clarify the nurse's specific responsibilities for what happens to patients.[3]

The heavy emphasis on life-saving responsibilities in nursing culture has affected the education of nurses in another important

[2] The patient's right to accept or to reject a recommended treatment which cannot be guaranteed to help him or to save his life is an assumption underlying sound medical practice. The doctor carries legal and moral responsibility for telling the patient his diagnosis and for explaining the limits of the therapeutic regimes which he proposes. Allowing patients opportunities to make these decisions is a serious responsibility in medical practice. See Frank J. Ayd, "The Hopeless Case," *Journal of the American Medical Association*, 181 (September 29, 1966), pp. 1099–1102.

[3] The assumption is made that responsibility cannot be delegated to another person unless concomitant authority is also delegated. More important, perhaps, responsibility must also be assumed. An individual cannot be forced to assume responsibility for his actions. The point is an important one and has relevance for nurses. In their work—whether it be in hospitals or in schools of nursing—the organization of activities provides for a dispersion of authority. Under these conditions, individuals can easily avoid assuming personal responsibility for their actions.

way. Teaching practices that stress the dangers of negligent performance encourage students to become overly concerned about making mistakes and may even discourage them from assuming responsibility for many of their actions. Perhaps the heavy reliance on hospital routines and ritualistic approaches by many practicing nurses has its origins in an early exposure to teachers or supervisors who were preoccupied—perhaps even panicked—by fears about negligence. There is a need to reverse the present tendency to emphasize the danger of making mistakes, and instead to foster a climate in which the reality of human error is recognized. The students need to learn ways of minimizing the possibility of making serious errors in practice, but they also need to be shown how to learn from their own failures. Nursing, like medicine, is a high-risk occupation, and the scope of nursing practice—particularly as it relates to medical practice—is undergoing change.[4] Whenever a situation is in flux, the choice of appropriate action may be unclear—thus the chance of an error in judgment increases.[5] The tendency to fix blame for mistakes can have a negative effect on the student's developing identity as a nurse. Students in nursing need help in recognizing that their actions as nurses are seldom all bad or all good, and that failures can serve as bases for growth and self-understanding.

The Idealization of Individual Responsibility for Patients

By and large, most nurse teachers place heavy stress on the individual nurse's responsibility for what happens to patients. In a sense this action reflects an idealization of the special-duty nurse of the past and maintains an image of bedside nursing despite the reality of what has happened to nursing practice in recent years.[6]

[4] See Nathan Hershey, "Scope of Nursing Practice," *American Journal of Nursing*, 66 (January, 1966), pp. 117–120.
[5] Richard J. Hill, "The Right to Fail," *Nursing Outlook*, 13 (April, 1965), p. 41.
[6] For a discussion of the persistence of the imagery of bedside nursing, see Anselm Strauss, "The Structure and Ideology of American Nursing," in Fred Davis, ed., *The Nursing Profession* (New York: Wiley, 1966), pp. 84–96.

Within the hospital, multiple numbers of nurses provide care for individual patients in most instances, and no one nurse carries complete responsibility for them. In practice, professional nurses often perform many managerial tasks and give direction to a wide variety of trained and untrained personnel. In addition, the technical activities within the hospital take precedence over the care activities, because the social and psychological aspects of patient care are not explicitly built into the hospital's accountability system.[7]

It would appear that teachers could take a more realistic approach to defining the specific responsibilities assumed by the professional nurse in the hospital. In addition, they need to consider whether the presently used patient assignment method with its one-to-one emphasis effectively prepares students for the problems they will encounter as practicing nurses.[8] Assignment innovations are certainly indicated if students are to be better prepared for the administrative and coordinating functions that comprise hospital nursing today. Talk about team nursing does not necessarily prepare students for the realities of hospital work.[9] If professional nurses are to be responsible for the activities performed by less well prepared hospital workers, then they need practice as students in delegating tasks and in supervising the outcomes.

One of the pressing needs is for teachers to counteract the present tendency to perpetuate the physician as being in the sole authority position, and to provide students with concrete direction in learning how to work effectively with physicians in the best interests of patients. Many difficulties faced by dying patients stem directly from lack of communication between doctors and nurses.

[7] Anselm L. Strauss, Barney Glaser, and Jeanne Quint, "The Non-accountability of Terminal Care," *Hospitals, J.A.H.A.*, 38 (January 16, 1964), pp. 73–74.

[8] Margaret Aasterud Williams, "Student Experiences in Working with Groups: Their Relevance to Nursing Service," *Nursing Forum*, Vol. 4, No. 4 (1965), pp. 76–82.

[9] Margaret Aasterud Williams, "The Myths and Assumptions About Team Nursing," *Nursing Forum*, Vol. 3, No. 4 (1964), pp. 61–73.

Although somewhat reluctantly, physicians themselves are beginning to recognize the nurse's contribution to patient welfare,

> Certainly the nurse's role as a go-between for physicians and patient is a perilous one and should not generally be required. Nevertheless, I think nurses should be a little bolder about reporting patients' questions and dissatisfactions to physicians. They may risk being called meddlesome, but I think we physicians need their help.[10]

Perhaps the peril can decrease as more physicians have the opportunity to work closely with nurses who do not withdraw from talking with them about the problems that interfere with patient well-being, including those problems inadvertently produced by the doctor himself. The students need assignments in which they can learn to communicate productively with physicians and can see how their actions contribute to positive results for the patients.

It is important to recognize that many of the communication problems between physicians and nurses stem directly from societal norms for male-female relationships—male dominance and assumed male superiority. The nurse's historical role of "handmaiden" serves to reinforce the subordinate female position and has been perpetuated in the minds of many practicing physicians.[11] Because most physicians are men and most nurses women, there is a real need for nursing and medical students to have opportunities to learn how to work together productively and to respect the differences in their contributions to patient care.

What the students are told is good nursing practice and what they see on the hospital wards often vary considerably. For one thing, the ward system is not organized to provide for the social and psychological needs of patients in the same way that it is organized to implement diagnostic and therapeutic procedures.

[10] Carl N. Brownsberger, "Emotional Stress Connected with Surgery," *Nursing Forum*, Vol. 4, No. 4 (1965), p. 55.

[11] For a discussion of this point, see Luther P. Christman, "Nurse-Physician Communications in the Hospital," *Journal of the American Medical Association*, 194 (November 1, 1965), p. 541.

Communication between physicians and nurses about the former types of patient problems does not usually occur on a regular basis.[12] Patients, perhaps especially those who are dying, often suffer the consequences. There is a real need for students to see practicing nurses, especially their teachers, actively engaged in initiating changes in nursing practice to offset the fragmenting effects that the hospital social structure creates for patient well-being.[13]

Conversation as a Component of Nursing Practice

By and large the conversational aspects of nursing practice have been presented to the students in generalized rather than specific terms, with a few exceptions. There has been an emphasis on using the doctor's authority position as a means of avoiding certain interactions with patients (actually, dying patients represent only one case of the general category of difficult patients). Some teachers have stressed the importance of encouraging patients to ventilate feelings without giving concomitant attention to the appropriateness or inappropriateness of such actions under particular sets of circumstances. In spite of increased teaching about psychological patient care, patients' needs continue to be described primarily in terms of the disease or the prescribed medical treatment. Their needs as human beings—both personal and social—have often lacked specificity with respect to the implications for nursing action. Because students (and nurses in general) are seldom held accountable for what they say to patients, each nurse is essentially free to develop her own idiosyncratic ways of talking with them. The results for dying patients may or may not be positive.

What is taught about nursing practice will continue to be

[12] Jeanne C. Quint, "Communications Problems Affecting Patient Care in Hospitals," *Journal of the American Medical Association*, 195 (January 3, 1966), pp. 36–37. See also Luther P. Christman, *op. cit.*, pp. 539–544.

[13] The complexity of the nurse's position and functions has been thoughtfully discussed by Hans O. Mauksch in "The Organizational Context of Nursing Practice," in Fred Davis, ed., *The Nursing Profession* (New York: Wiley, 1966), pp. 107–137.

narrow in scope until there is a much broader base in behavioral science content. Further, there is a need for a specific clarification of the responsibilities the individual nurse can carry for the well-being of individual patients. The general notions about providing psychological nursing care are not very concrete with respect to either their substantive or their temporal dimensions and may well remain so until patient-centered research by nurses has been expanded.[14] Even with these limitations, however, students need to be helped to develop a more realistic appraisal of the nurse's responsibilities for patient well-being.[15]

Notwithstanding the important part played by nurses in implementing successful medical therapies, there is a need to consider more explicitly the particular ways in which nurses can help patients cope with the personal and social problems rising out of the dying situation. Much that nurses can offer to dying patients and their families is possible because of the context in which they meet, but nurses do not necessarily recognize how they can help. To that end there is a need for nurse students to participate in educational experiences that center directly on the nurse's responsibility for patient well-being. Undoubtedly these experiences should include exploring the patient's rights as a person, the limits of nursing practice, the effect of hospital social structure on what happens to patients, and other related matters. In a more specific sense, some discussions should be concerned solely with the dying patient. The students need to consider how and when they define patients as dying. The teachers need to help the students to understand the critical stages which the dying person faces as he moves toward the end of his life, and to consider how decisions and

[14] A progressive isolation, specifically with respect to talking about cancer and the possibility of dying, was one of the outcomes for women following mastectomy. In addition, the points of maximum social and psychological stress encountered during the first year following surgery followed a similar timing pattern. See Jeanne C. Quint, "Mastectomy—Symbol of Cure or Warning Sign?" GP, 29 (March, 1964), pp. 119–124.

[15] The phrase *patient well-being* rather than *patient care* is purposely used to indicate that we are here dealing primarily with human rather than medical matters.

actions by nurses greatly affect what happens to him. Through all of this, the teachers need to be aware of the emotional involvement that students face in learning how to provide comforting care for dying patients. Especially do the students need help in learning how to converse with patients when the latter want to talk openly about their approaching death.

Nurses are not generally aware that their conversations with dying patients are crucial events, often affecting the patients' lives in very significant ways. Furthermore, nurses have tended to abnegate their responsibilities for patient well-being by using the doctor's authority position as a protective shield—but patients have suffered as a result. What nurses have learned to do reflects the values, beliefs, and practices of nursing culture. If the values and beliefs underlying nursing practice are no longer in the best interests of patients, then educational programs that prepare nurses as practitioners are in need of revision. Those interested in change need to be aware that what happens to students during the first year in school plays a crucial part in the development of their identities as nurses.

Some Proposals for Change

The First Year in School

In talking with students and in analyzing their descriptions of and reactions to patients at different points in time, one is struck by the relative importance of first-year experiences in the development of basic attitudes toward dying patients. The lack of well-planned and coordinated teaching programs centered specifically on the nursing care of dying patients contributes to an environment in which many nursing students develop stereotyped and somewhat negative attitudes toward these patients. There is a tendency to perpetuate traditional nurse behavior patterns which students observe on the hospital wards, and often the practice of withdrawal from dying patients is quite well established by the end of the first year in school.

In my view, there is a need for change in what is taught about nursing practice and the care of dying patients. Basic to this change is the development of a well-planned and coordinated teaching program in which special attention is given to planning for the first year of study. There are both philosophic and pragmatic issues to be considered in the development of such a program. As a starting point, the substance of what is taught about death and dying needs to be expanded in at least two ways. Much more content about death as related to cultural patterns and societal values needs to be incorporated into the curriculum, and used as a basis for discussion. The present emphasis on practice *per se* needs to be expanded to give greater attention to the philosophic basis underlying nursing practice.[16]

Open discussions based on these content areas ought to begin before the students are assigned to patients. Such discussions can be one means for helping the students, most of whom have had little direct contact with dying, take a look at a practice problem that they will not find easy. Explorations of dying at the intellectual level may well serve as rehearsals for some of the concrete realities and emotional difficulties that students are likely to face when they are assigned to dying patients.[17] With or without rehearsals many students become personally uncomfortable during assignments to dying patients because the experiences stir up their own anxieties about death. Class discussions about death are of limited value without concomitant planning for first assignments to dying patients under conditions that maximize the chances for positive outcomes for the students.

Another important need is for class discussions in which teachers and students talk openly about decision making and nursing practice. These discussions will not provide easy answers to nursing problems, but they are essential if students are to understand the kinds of decisions that nursing work requires. The students need

---

[16] For one nurse's viewpoint, see Lorraine Olszewski, "A Philosophy of Nursing Care," *Nursing Forum*, Vol. 4, No. 4 (1965), pp. 32–35.

[17] The positive value of this approach has been suggested by Berniece M. Wagner, "Teaching Students to Work with the Dying," *American Journal of Nursing*, 64 (November, 1964), pp. 128–131.

to explore for themselves what is meant by life-death decision making. They need the chance to discuss the many issues involved in actions taken to prolong life, or to shorten life. Class sessions on these matters would have added value if both nursing and medical students were participants. Joint classes would have several positive effects. They would provide opportunity for the two groups of students to explore together some of the serious issues and difficult problems they will have in common as health practitioners.[18] Open and free discussions about these matters would also provide practice in exchanging ideas and in learning how to work together in a more productive way.

Many nursing students are unsure of themselves in talking with physicians, whom they tend to endow with extraordinary powers and abilities. Sometimes this uncertainty is reinforced by encounters on the wards with physicians who respond to the students in a brusque or critical manner. The joint discussions described above might well provide these young women with the chance to learn how to discuss and solve patient-care problems with medical practitioners, albeit future ones, in a discussion situation—the classroom—removed from the threats of actual practice. Furthermore, the medical students would have the chance to hear the nurses' viewpoints on patient problems and to learn how the mutual exchange of information could lessen misunderstanding and thereby contribute to better care for dying patients.

The classroom can be exceedingly useful for helping the nurse student learn about many aspects of death and dying. It cannot replace the patient assignment as a direct experience in learning how to function as a nurse in the presence of death or dying.

The Use of Patients as School Assignments

When schools of nursing do not provide for systematic and planned assignments to dying patients, or expose the students to

---

[18] A secondary analysis of field notes by Anselm Strauss from a study of the University of Kansas Medical School indicates that medical students have very little if any of this type of discussion with their teachers. See Howard S. Becker, et al., *Boys in White* (Chicago: University of Chicago Press, 1961).

death under relatively controlled conditions, two major results are possible. The faculty-controlled laboratory pattern can lead to *no* assignments for some students, when care of the dying is not explicitly built into the assignment plan. By comparison, the hospital-work type of assignment tends to produce chance encounters with death and dying under widely varying assignment conditions. The outcomes for students are not always predictable, but there is a relatively high probability that some students will have bad experiences that will foster a retreat from dying patients —again reinforcing the general cultural pattern of withdrawal from these persons. Under either assignment plan, there is the possibility that some students will have overwhelming encounters with dying patients before the students are able to cope with the specific assignment expectations.

These findings suggest that students can be better prepared for later assignments to dying patients if they are exposed to death early and in a well-planned way. This exposure needs to be both observational and participative. In my opinion, nurse students can well profit from observational assignments to death situations, preceded and followed by class discussions with their teachers, as part of their early orientation to nursing practice. By eliminating any practice responsibilities and by providing for open discussion, observational assignments under reasonably controlled circumstances can buffer some of the shock reactions associated with uncontrolled first-time encounters with death. As preparation, the observation assignments might well be preceded by a period of concentrated reading and class discussion focused on death as a hospital event. These observations could serve the valuable function of bringing the students into direct contact with death and dying without the pressures of nursing practice responsibilities.

The students can see death and talk about what they see, but they also need the chance to participate as nurses in performing the tasks associated with death and dying. To that end each student needs to have the experience of providing postmortem body care under conditions that provide her with support and encouragement and minimize the possibilities of a traumatic aftermath. Support is probably best provided when the student shares nurse responsibility with another person (preferably a teacher) who is both experienced as a nurse and sensitive to newcomer reactions to death. To minimize the impact of factors of social loss, it would be best for these initial encounters with death to be on a geriatrics ward, and a pediatric setting should not be used until later.

Implementation of an effective teaching program on care of the dying requires well-prepared teachers and a system for coordinating the use of patients as assignments. The first-year faculty, in particular, ought to be highly sensitive nurses who are themselves relatively comfortable with their own feelings about death and dying and able to talk freely with the students about the various issues involved in providing care for dying patients. The teachers need to be cognizant of the hazardous aspects of patient assignments.[19] Further, they need to be aware of the influence they bring to bear on the situation through rehearsal (or nonrehearsal) with the students in preparation for these assignments, and through accountability (or nonaccountability) for reporting back during and after the assignments. By being aware of their own expectations, the teachers can make better use of early assignments to dying patients to help the students prepare for later meetings with more complex assignments. There could be value in the student watching the teacher, rather than the reverse, during some of these initial assignments.[20] The students might learn a great deal by observing their teachers in action and by engaging in a give-and-take discussion with them afterward about what they did and why. Indeed, the most profitable learning might come from discussions in which the teachers openly talk about the pros and cons of their own actions and of the reasons underlying their choices. Conceivably, the students could have very positive experiences in knowing that their teachers were subject to errors in judgment

[19] Jeanne C. Quint, "The Hidden Hazards in Patient Assignments," *Nursing Outlook*, 13 (November, 1965), pp. 50–54.

[20] This idea was suggested by Dorothy M. Smith, Dean of the College of Nursing and Chief of Nursing Practice, The J. Hillis Health Center, University of Florida, Gainesville, in a letter to the author.

but could use these errors as means for improving their own practices as nurses.

There is also need for a coordinated assignment program that would minimize the chances for any one student to have an overwhelming assignment with its untoward consequences. This program would require careful planning, particularly for patient assignments during the first year in school. Undoubtedly, one person would have to carry responsibility for organizing the program and for facilitating communication among the various teachers concerned. The problem is not solely that of ensuring that students are assigned to dying patients but rather of providing an environment in which students can learn to recognize many situations in which death may be of critical importance to the patient. For example, during periods of uncertainty—such as prior to major surgery—some patients may get feelings of personal security simply by being able to talk openly with a nurse about the possibility of dying, or their fears that this might happen.

Identity Stress: The Emotional Impact of Dying

There can be little doubt of the emotional impact on the student of encounters with dying patients. Often assignments to these patients precipitate feelings of helplessness, frustration, and hopelessness. There is certainly a need for a school environment in which the student can confront her feelings directly, rather than pushing them aside and avoiding patient situations which precipitate similar reactions. Such a supporting environment is crucial during the first year in school when many students are being exposed to illness and death and hospital life for the first time. The students need teachers who can provide them with support and direction as they learn how to perform the many activities that comprise nursing practice.

In particular, the students need practice in letting patients talk about topics which cause them, the students, to feel uncomfortable. To develop this skill, they need a teacher who can let them talk about the difficulties that they encounter during these conversations with patients.[21] The teacher can provide one kind of support by listening and by allowing the students to express feelings engendered during the conversations with patients. The teacher can also provide another kind of support—that of direction—by assisting the student to understand the context of interaction with the patient and to speculate about actions to be taken in the future. The process of learning how to provide compassionate care in situations containing high emotional risk for the self (including the whens, whats, and hows of talking about tension-producing topics) is time-consuming and far from easy. It requires nurse teachers who are sensitive and perceptive and knowledgeable about human behavior and about what happens to patients in hospitals.

This kind of teaching is far from simple. The nurse instructors who assume responsibility for it will undoubtedly need support and direction themselves—particularly in the beginning. It is here that the services of persons from other disciplines—psychiatry, psychology, the social sciences—may well play a major part in helping the faculty develop "backstopping" techniques for themselves as well as for the students.[22] These specialists can also be used as consultants in the application of behavioral science content to the practice of nursing. However, decisions about what constitutes responsible nursing practice must be made by nurses themselves.

Some patient assignments are more difficult than others for the students to face. Being around a child with a fatal illness, for example, is notably upsetting to most. Support and direction from the teacher are crucially important during these assignments be-

21 Pamela A. Holsclaw in "Nursing in High Emotional Risk Areas," *Nursing Forum*, Vol. 4, No. 4 (1965), pp. 36–45, suggests that in order for the nurse to offer sympathetic and compassionate care to a patient she must go through the experience of facing her anxiety about such threats as the fact that people die, and must learn to utilize her own defenses in a way that is constructive rather than destructive for patients. This process of change requires support from another person.

22 The need for support in carrying on in the face of a difficult task is described by Edna Mae Jones, "Who Supports the Nurse?" *Nursing Outlook*, 10 (July, 1962), pp. 476–478.

cause the patient situation has several factors contributing to emotional distress for the student. In fact, a carefully guided training experience is probably essential for the nurse who wants to specialize in pediatrics.[23]

Some assignments are difficult because of the technical procedures the student is expected to perform. The teacher can help the student by being aware of these difficulties, for beginning students in particular, and by watching for indications that a student is being overwhelmed by the assignment expectations. When stresses of this nature appear, the teacher is often in a position to offer guidance and help—sometimes even by taking over parts of the assignment the student finds impossible to perform well. Undoubtedly, the teacher can contribute to student well-being by selecting assignments that are challenging without being overpowering. It is also well to recognize that students can be overwhelmed by other factors that are shocking or disconcerting. Intense pain, sloughing skin, or bizarre behavior are among the many aspects of the patient assignment that may be troublesome for students. They need help and understanding while learning how to provide comforting care under such circumstances. Effective teaching requires instructors who are relatively comfortable with these and many other problems of dying patients.

The Level of Teacher Preparation

In general, nurse teachers are not well prepared to teach about the care of dying patients because they are not themselves comfortable with many nursing problems associated with death. Thus, many tend to perpetuate the traditional ways used by nurses to avoid the problem, though often they do so unintentionally. Also, the organization of the school of nursing is such that individual teachers can often successfully evade contact with dying because teaching about death—or rather about specific aspects of death as a nursing problem—has not been specifically delegated. The teachers often are not held accountable for many aspects of what

[23] See Florence Erickson, "The Need for a Specialist in Modern Pediatric Nursing," *Nursing Forum*, 4 (1965), pp. 24–31.

they do—in this instance, what they teach (or do not teach) about death and dying.

The problem is not to establish a rigid pattern of accountability for those who are teaching, but to clarify the specific responsibilities which different teachers carry for teaching about death and to ensure that the students obtain those patient assignments that are deemed essential. Assignments to patients who are dying fall into the essential category.

As a consequence of changes in graduate education in nursing, many new teachers are learning how to be effective in helping students during tension-producing patient assignments. These teachers are bringing new perspectives to established faculties (and to students, too), but their ideas are sometimes met with resistance by those who have been teaching for some time. Thus, the effect on the teaching program as a whole may be minimal.

The new teachers may not necessarily be well prepared to teach about care of the dying, either in the classroom or on the hospital wards. However, some are bringing a sharpened and sensitive approach to helping students with this difficult nursing problem. Also, seasoned nurse teachers who have learned, usually through personal experiences with death, to guide students skillfully through difficult assignments to dying patients are often handicapped by a limited perspective of nursing which blocks them from developing a broader perspective on the problem of dying. Even the best-prepared teachers might find value in a reorientation program that gives particular attention to the changing responsibilities posed for nurses by technological advances and by social innovations. Certainly there is a need for less-well-prepared teachers to be helped in learning how to be more effective in teaching the care of dying patients.

One way to get better preparation is to return to school for advanced study, but not all nurse teachers can take this step. Another way might be to offer a concentrated summer workshop centered specifically on death as a nursing problem. This workshop could be developed for teachers from many different schools and offered at a central location. It might also be offered to individual faculties and conducted within their own institutions. In either case the program ought to include patient assignments under close supervision in addition to extensive reading and discussion about the cultural, social, and behavioral aspects of dying. In a sense, the teachers have to go through the painful experience of seeing how old patterns of practice get in the way of providing effective care for dying patients and effective teaching for students.

The difficulties involved in helping teachers of nursing to change their attitudes and practices with respect to dying patients should not be underestimated.[24] The process of changing already set ways of behaving around dying patients and their families is a difficult and emotionally disturbing process. Like others, teachers of nursing are bound to resist changes that threaten their basic identities.

Counteracting the Retreat from Hospital Work

My findings suggest that the students who are best prepared to provide good psychological care for patients tend to retreat from hospital work because they have limited chances to gain personal satisfaction in the work.[25] The education of psychologically oriented nurses seems like a fruitless venture unless steps can also be taken to alter the hospital social structure so as to provide opportunities for these persons to make their skills available to the patients. This may require the creation of new nursing positions; it may mean experimentation with novel ways of providing continuity of experience for hospitalized patients.[26] The need for innovation in nursing practices and in the organization of nursing services is, perhaps, most needed in teaching hospitals, where patients can easily feel lost in the confusion and complexity of a

[24] Jeanne C. Quint, "Some Problems in Applying the Findings of Research," *Nursing Outlook*, 13 (August, 1965), p. 53.

[25] This notion is confirmed by Fred Davis, Virginia L. Olesen, and Elvi Waik Whittaker in, "Problems and Issues in Collegiate Nursing Education," in Fred Davis, ed., *The Nursing Profession* (New York: Wiley, 1966), pp. 162–167.

[26] See Doris O'Connor and Faye Hagan, "Liaison Nurse," *American Journal of Nursing*, 64 (June, 1964), pp. 101–103; and Helen G. Wolford, "Complemental Nursing Care and Practice," *Nursing Forum*, Vol. 3, No. 1 (1964), pp. 8–20.

large multipurpose institution.[27] Clearly, faculties of schools of nursing would serve as better models of professional nurses if they assumed more direct responsibility for initiating changes in the practice of nursing.

As far as improving care for the dying is concerned, there is much that can be done by nurses in hospitals *if* they are willing to assume responsibility for the well-being of these patients. There is a real need for those in charge of nursing services in hospitals to recognize how current assignment practices often contribute to less than satisfactory outcomes both for those who are dying and for the nursing staff. For innovation to take place, two steps appear to be necessary: involvement of the medical staff in cooperative planning for better services to dying patients and provision of support and guidance on a regular basis to the nursing staff directly involved in providing care for patients.[28] Nurses on the wards are in a position to provide compassionate care to those who are dying if nurse administrators are prepared to allow this kind of functioning and can provide the environment in which it is possible. However, the difficulties involved in changing well-established hospital practices should not be underestimated. As Holsclaw has observed,

> If these defenses are as well institutionalized as these studies indicate, nursing service cannot be expected to suddenly provide support to nurses in areas where high emotional risk initially stimulated the system.[29]

There are, to be sure, hospitals in which nurses are already working to improve the care they give to dying patients.[30] Nursing educators and nursing service administrators might well combine forces to work toward achieving a similar goal in many hospitals.

The general practice of not being very open with the patient

[27] One approach to this problem is offered by Dorothy M. Smith in "Nursing Education and Nursing Service," *Journal of the American Medical Association*, 191 (February 1, 1965), pp. 416–418.

[28] Jeanne C. Quint, "Nursing Services and the Care of Dying Patients: Some Speculations," *Nursing Science*, 2 (December, 1964), pp. 432–443.

[29] Holsclaw, *op. cit.*, p. 43.

[30] Ramona Powell Davidson, "To Give Care in Terminal Illness," *American Journal of Nursing*, 66 (January, 1966), pp. 74–75.

about his own dying is a cultural phenomenon reflecting a wish to deny the reality of death. As a consequence, the patient's right to shape his own way of living—and dying—has sometimes been assumed by others. Allowing dying patients more opportunities to participate openly in their own dying is a serious and difficult problem, one for which nurses, doctors, and laymen in this society have not been well prepared. Clearly, nurses need to be aware that assuming responsibility for the well-being of dying patients in hospitals is a risky enterprise because it requires altering some well-established hospital and nursing practices. Clearly, too, presently existing practices in hospitals are unlikely to be changed by the efforts of nurses alone. Changes in hospital policies and practices must be sanctioned by higher authorities—the boards of directors and the medical staffs of hospitals—and, ultimately, be accepted by the public being served. Yet nurses can assume leadership in initiating change by accepting responsibility for helping the dying patient share in the decisions affecting how he will live and how he will die.[31]

In Conclusion

If the care of dying patients is to have a more rational and systematic base, then education of those in the health professions with respect to this care is of critical importance. The problem is not solely a nursing problem, but schools of nursing can do a great deal to change the situation that presently exists. Professional

---

[31] Assuming this responsibility for dying patients should not be construed as taking over the physician's responsibility for telling the patient his diagnosis and prognosis. Rather it means the nurse's responsibility for the dying patient requires a delicate balance between making decisions for the patient (when he is unable to do so for himself) and providing him opportunities to decide matters which are clearly his own to decide. This responsibility also means interceding on the patient's behalf with others (physicians, families, friends, clergy, other nurses) when he is unable to manage these interactions on his own. See Jeanne C. Quint, "Institutionalized Practices of Information Control," *Psychiatry*, 28 (May, 1965), pp. 129–132. Another way of viewing the nurse's responsibility for patients is given by Sister Madeleine Clemence in "Existentialism: A Philosophy of Commitment," *American Journal of Nursing*, 66 (March, 1966), pp. 500–505.

nurses often hold positions in which they could assume considerable responsibility for the well-being of dying patients and their families, but nurses have not been prepared for this kind of responsibility. This chapter contains some proposals that might lead in that direction. They are offered in full recognition that change would not be easy to effect. The problem is that of helping young people understand how deep-seated societal values—in this instance attitudes toward death—influence their effectiveness as professional practitioners.

Teaching innovation requires faculties who recognize the need for a rational and systematic educational approach to a serious professional problem. No easy solution is available. Any faculty willing to initiate change will have to decide when and how to start and where to get help with the practical problems they will face. Certainly, nurses who are willing to assume new responsibilities should be prepared to encounter difficulties along the way. For one thing, breaking old, established patterns of working with physicians is bound to be threatening to many doctors, especially those who tend to think of nurses in terms of "the good old days." Nurse teachers should not be surprised when their efforts to initiate change are misinterpreted and misunderstood. Rather they might anticipate these responses by enlisting advance support from those physicians who recognize and appreciate the need for coordinated services for hospitalized patients.

As this study has shown, students are easily upset by assignments that cause them to feel helpless and hopeless. Those who work through these feelings apparently must go through periods of depression and anger. Nurse teachers need to be aware that these reactions are normal to the learning process. Changing attitudes is a time-consuming and difficult matter. The teachers can also expect that the students will sometimes use poor judgment or make conversational *faux pas* as they learn how to interact with the patients and their families. Schematic knowledge about the grief process can quite easily be presented in the abstract.[32] Pro-

[32] George L. Engel, "Grief and Grieving," *American Journal of Nursing*, **64** (September, 1964), pp. 93–98.

viding students with direction and support while they are actively putting these ideas into practice is quite a different matter.

There are many serious issues which need to be openly discussed by those who are teaching. There are new ways of keeping people alive for longer periods of time, and these changes greatly affect nursing practices and decisions in the hospital. If students are to learn to accept more responsibility for what happens to dying patients, for example, interceding with the physician on behalf of the patient, then students must be helped to move away from looking to the doctor for direction. To do so requires the development of a philosophy of nursing practice in which the patient's rights are clearly understood and the nurse's responsibilities involve more than simply carrying out the doctor's written orders.

The hospital has become a very complex enterprise, and the patient can easily become lost amidst the confusion of personnel attending him. The dying patient—the forgotten man in the hospital—can well use an ally whose goal is to help him live with his human problems, and the personal and social strains associated with his outcast position.[33] The professional nurse can assume this function if she is willing to accept the risks of moving into new kinds of role relationships with physicians, patients, families, and all manner of professional and nonprofessional hospital workers. This is a solemn responsibility because it means moving out of the traditional nurse role with its emphasis on delegated medical tasks and comfort care into a more active role in which communicating with and on behalf of patients becomes a primary concern. This recommendation in no way negates the importance of providing physical comfort and implementing diagnostic and therapeutic procedures. Rather it implies that patients can also benefit from the services of well-prepared psychologically oriented nurses who provide them with continuity of contact and serve as liaisons between them and many other persons.

Obviously the changes suggested earlier in this chapter cannot all be started simultaneously. In fact, many of the recommenda-

[33] Caught up in feelings of guilt and grief, the family may add to his isolation.

tions can only come about when nursing faculties are better prepared to teach about the care of dying patients and to serve as models for the students to see in action. A first priority, then, is to educate nurse teachers for the task. This involves two goals: providing assistance to those who are already teaching and strengthening the programs offered to new teachers in graduate school. Without a concentrated effort in both directions, little change can be expected in the preparation of nursing practitioners.

A second priority is to provide nurses in hospitals with direct assistance in meeting the problems they encounter with dying patients. There is tremendous need for staff development programs with respect to this problem. Nursing faculties could well provide assistance by helping hospital nurses in the development of conferences and workshops and in finding resource personnel from other disciplines (clergymen, psychologists, psychiatrists, sociologists, educators). One of the pressing needs in hospitals is to find ways of helping the nursing staff to obtain greater satisfaction from their assignments to dying patients.

It would be impossible to initiate all the changes proposed in this chapter without a radical impact on nursing and on hospital care. Implicitly, many questions have been raised which go far beyond the care of dying patients. One fundamental issue is concerned with how to balance professional decisions in the best interests of patients with the patient's rights to know and to decide matters for himself.[34] Nurses as well as doctors face many patient situations in which this judgment is required, and they are likely to encounter even more as diagnostic and treatment techniques increase in complexity. The education of both groups has given far more attention to the physical sciences and technical aspects

[34] The seriousness of this issue with respect to advancing medical technology has recently been discussed in several nonprofessional publications: Francis D. Moore, "Ethics in New Medicine: Tissue Transplants," *The Nation* (April 5, 1965), pp. 358–362; Albert Rosenfield, "Will Man Direct His Own Revolution?" *Life* (October 1, 1965), pp. 96–109; John Lear, "Do We Need New Rules for Experimenting on People?" *Saturday Review* (February 5, 1966), pp. 61–70.

of practice than to the behavioral sciences and their application to professional practice.

Perhaps the most critical question raised by this study has to do with educational preparation of nurses for all the stress-producing problems that they meet as practitioners. From the relative protection of middle-class American life, many beginning nurses quite abruptly find themselves in a world full to overflowing with emotionally disturbing events and activities. Just as encounters with death can produce shock reactions with far-reaching consequences, so also do encounters with disfigurement and crippling, with human suffering and agonizing pain. On entering nursing, young women are expected to perform many tasks of an intimate nature on the bodies of other persons. The Williams [35] found that students did not anticipate the intimate physical contacts which many nursing activities required, nor were they prepared for the drastic emotional shock associated with such patient care problems as urination, defecation, soiled linens, distasteful odors, and patient-family reactions to pain and death. Also, the students were often emotionally disturbed when they had to view or handle body parts, disfigurements, or the genitals of their patients. In fact, the first year in nursing school is one of intense identity stress and value confusion as students come face to face with many situations in which their personal values are at stake.

Nursing is an occupation concerned with many tension-producing aspects of living. Yet the evidence presented in this book indicates that the socialization techniques utilized by nursing faculties do not make sufficient allowance for the emotional conflicts that many young people experience in the process of becoming nurses. The transition to nursing brings young Americans into close proximity with all manner of social situations which threaten deep-seated cultural values and attitudes. It is not solely death that causes emotional distress and personal conflicts of a serious nature. If the first year in school is indeed a critical tran-

[35] Thomas Rhys Williams and Margaret M. Williams, "The Socialization of the Student Nurse," *Nursing Research*, 8 (Winter, 1959), p. 22.

sition period in the process of becoming a nurse, then the need is great for faculties to be aware of the serious human problems encountered by students as they live through the experience.

The basic problem is that of providing an environment in which the students can recognize how many of their attitudes, acquired through acculturation in the wider society, seriously affect their actions as professional practitioners and interfere with their abilities to provide compassionate and understanding care. It is no simple matter to show human concern for a patient whose looks, actions, condition, or background are threatening to one's basic system of values—thus to one's sense of identity, as a person or a nurse. The educational changes proposed earlier have implications that reach far beyond the care of dying patients.

Appendix A | Study Background
and Methods

The data on which this book is based were
collected as part of an extensive sociological investigation of dying in hospitals. Begun in 1961, the overall project focused on
understanding dying as a social phenomenon with consequences
for the hospital and its staff as well as for the patients and their
families. Toward that end, a body of fieldwork data was collected
in several different hospitals over a three-year period.[1] The project had been in progress for over a year when I began to study
the problem of how students of nursing learn about dying pa-

[1] For a more extensive discussion of the collection and analysis of field-
work data, see Barney G. Glaser and Anselm L. Strauss, "Discovery of Sub-
stantive Theory: A Basic Strategy Underlying Qualitative Research," *The
American Behavioral Scientist*, 8 (February, 1965), pp. 5–12; Barney G.
Glaser, "The Constant Comparative Method of Qualitative Analysis," *Social
Problems* 12 (Spring, 1965), pp. 436–445; Barney G. Glaser and Anselm
L. Strauss, *Awareness of Dying* (Chicago: Aldine, 1965), pp. 286–293; and
Barney G. Glaser and Anselm L. Strauss, "The Purpose and Credibility of
Qualitative Research," *Nursing Research*, 15 (Winter, 1966), pp. 56–61.

tients. Many variables and relationships had already been established, and thus influenced both the collection and the analysis of these data.[2]

The fieldwork data indicated that what nurses do when they work around dying patients in the hospital varies with the social relationships and work demands of different ward settings. However, nurses bring to this work some expectations and behavior patterns that were formed while they were students of nursing. Interest in learning how this process came about was stimulated by conversations with newly graduated nurses from many parts of the United States.[3] These young women reported wide variations in their encounters with death as students. Yet they showed many similarities in their attitudes and actions toward dying patients. This situation caused me to wonder how the instructional programs offered by schools of nursing led to these results. The problem became one of discovering *what* nurse students learned about death as a problem they would face in practice, *how* they learned it, and *when*. With this goal in mind, fieldwork and interview data were collected over a period of roughly three years. Five schools of nursing in the Bay Area of San Francisco served as primary sources for data gathering.

The Schools

The participating schools were similar in that graduates of the instructional programs were then eligible for licensure as registered nurses after satisfactory completion of a state examination. However, the five schools were chosen because they were dissimilar in several ways and thus could be studied comparatively. The

---

[2] For example, the concept of social loss (see Chapter 4, pp. 101–103) was developed as an explanatory variable for describing the reactions of hospital staff and others to the deaths of certain categories of patients. It was readily applicable to the reactions of nurse students to the same patient categories.

[3] These nurses either were or were eligible to become registered nurses. They were graduates of programs which varied in length (two to five years) and were administered by different institutions (junior colleges, hospitals, senior colleges, and universities).

schools were selected because of their different administrative and organizational patterns and because they used different kinds of hospitals for practice. I was thereby able to study what happened to the students under different sets of structural conditions.

One school was administered by a university and offered a program leading to the baccalaureate degree. The school was situated on a medical center campus, and students in the undergraduate program completed two years of college work before taking the three-year nursing curriculum. The school also offered an undergraduate curriculum leading to the baccalaureate degree for registered nurses, as well as graduate curricula at the masters and post-masters levels of education. During the 1962–1963 years when data collection began, the undergraduate students in the fundamentals of nursing course were divided into three groups, one control and two experimental. Different teaching approaches to the development of observation skills were applied to each group. The students were then tested for the influence of these different approaches on the procedural skills developed by them during each semester. Although these were not incorporated into the experimental teaching program itself, the teachers of fundamentals also used settings other than medical and surgical wards for the first time. Some students had experiences on pediatrics wards, others in psychiatric settings, and some visited a family every three weeks. The three groups of faculty were drawn from the four nursing areas, and in addition there were some who had taught the fundamentals course previously.[4]

Another assignment variation was used in the maternal-child nursing course given during the second year. Each student was assigned to a family for the full semester. The focus was to assist the students in identifying varying kinds of stress situations encountered during the child rearing and childbearing periods. The faculty used one hour of individual conferences weekly

[4] Report of Curriculum Evaluation 1959–1963, submitted to the Collegiate Board of Review, Department of Baccalaureate and Higher Degree Programs, National League for Nursing (September 1, 1963), pp. 15–21.

for talking about these families with the students.[5] (Data from interviews showed that the prolonged contact required by these assignments provided intense stress situations for some students who became involved and overidentified with some of their families' problems.)

The medical center campus also provided facilities for schools of dentistry, medicine, and pharmacy. Two teaching hospitals and a neuropsychiatric institute were available to these schools for teaching and research purposes. At the time of the study the school of nursing used these institutions as principal resources for hospital assignments. To a limited extent assignments were made in a county hospital and a veterans' administration hospital by those teaching the fundamentals of nursing course. During the third year, students had assignments in a variety of public health agencies as well as in hospitals.

The other four schools were administered by hospitals and offered three-year instructional programs. Two of the schools were organized as separate departments within the hospital organization. Both of these hospitals were private nonprofit institutions, one under the auspices of the Roman Catholic Church and the other incorporated under the auspices of the Episcopal Church. In the remaining two schools, the director of nursing held a joint appointment as administrator for both the school of nursing and the department of nursing service. One of these schools was affiliated with a private nonsectarian hospital, the other with a county hospital.

With one exception each of the hospital schools used a local college for courses in the biological and behavioral sciences and, sometimes, for other non-nursing courses. Although all utilized more than one hospital for school assignments, the bulk of student experience with patients was provided in the school's home hospital. During the period of data collection the schools offered relatively stable educational programs except for one school which was initiating major revisions in the curriculum. Only one school

[5] *Ibid.*, pp. 22–23.

(the Roman Catholic) included religious teaching as a regular part of the curriculum.

Three of the schools had student bodies that were roughly equivalent in size, but they differed somewhat in the numbers of nursing instructors who were on the faculty.[6] School B had eighty-two students and nine full-time nursing teachers. School C had seventy-three students and ten teachers. School D had ninety-one students and five teachers of nursing. Somewhat larger in size, School E had a student body of 150 with eleven full-time nurse faculty members. (School A, the university school, had 124 basic undergraduate students, and twenty-two teachers were assigned to the undergraduate curriculum.) On the average, the university students were two years older than the others, many of whom enrolled in nursing school shortly after graduation from high school.

Consideration was given to collecting data from students enrolled in a two-year nursing curriculum conducted under the auspices of a junior college. After several interviews with students in each of the participating schools, I decided that there was little likelihood of discovering different or unusual findings from such interviews because the circumstances under which students in two-year programs were assigned to patients were not unlike those already under scrutiny.

The Research Methods

The research design reflected the exploratory nature of the inquiry and the sociological orientation of the researcher. Research methods were chosen to provide for flexibility of approach and to maximize the comparative value of the data obtained. I was seeking to understand what happened to nurse students within the framework of the school's instructional program, but not what happened in terms of quantity (i.e., counting the numbers of students having particular kinds of experiences). Rather, I

[6] Enrollment and faculty figures are for the 1962–1963 year. Excluded from faculty counts are those holding administrative positions in the school or dual positions (teaching supervisors).

was concerned with clarifying the kinds of incidents which took place, the circumstances surrounding them, and the immediate and long-term results of these experiences. The study did not begin with a clear-cut set of hypotheses and highly structured data-gathering instruments. Instead the approach was an open one to allow for the discovery of variables and a systematic formulation of their interrelationships. The collection of data began with a period of preliminary fieldwork and interviewing at the medical center teaching hospital. Fieldwork thereafter became only a subsidiary method and interviewing became the major method for collecting data. (My activities as a fieldworker were not restricted to collecting data about students. The project as a whole was concerned with many questions relevant to dying in hospitals, and I collected fieldwork data germane to a variety of different problems in which dying was a central issue.)

Preliminary Fieldwork

My initial conversations were with young staff nurses who had been out of nursing school for less than six months. The names of these young women were obtained through the director of nursing. The interviews were arranged by me through face-to-face contact with the nurses and were conducted on the wards where they were assigned. The interviews were collected on tape, with additional observations and more casual conversations recorded by me as field notes. The nurses were working on several different wards which provided services for patients with medical or surgical problems.

At the same time, I talked with several teachers in the school of nursing as a means of establishing contacts with the students. Arrangements were made to attend classes to ask for volunteers to be interviewed. This technique did not prove to be particularly successful because only a few "brave" students offered their services, and these were not students who had had or were going through experiences involving dying patients. The strategy did serve as a starting point for contacting other students whose experiences were mentioned by the interviewees. School had just begun, and I was particularly interested in contacting students who were just starting their patient assignments. However, I also wanted to talk with those in their second and third years, as well as with some who were enrolled in different nursing courses. Thus the strategy of studying several comparison groups simultaneously was instituted during the preliminary data-gathering period.

My prior experience as a nurse and as a teacher of nurses, in both hospital and university schools of nursing, was extremely useful in helping me to decide when, where, and how to contact the students, their teachers, and members of the hospital staff. In addition, this background made it possible for me to converse easily with nurses and with students because their problems and concerns were familiar to me—I had been there once myself. I had also had intense and difficult personal and professional experiences with death and dying, and had developed an ability to talk about these subjects and to listen to others talk about personally meaningful experiences of a tension-producing nature. Just prior to joining the project staff, I had served as project director for a study of the adjustment problems faced by women with cancer. The experience of interviewing them about their fears and concerns ably prepared me for talking with nurse students about many kinds of incidents, including those which reactivated feelings of emotional upset during the retelling process.[7] Listening to these young women talk about some of the incidents was not always easy, as I shall indicate later.

My contacts with the students whom I interviewed came about in various ways. From the teachers I learned where the students were assigned in the hospital, and I began to circulate on these wards and to chat with the students and the staff. These conversations told me which students were assigned to dying pa-

[7] For a discussion of some of the difficulties encountered in collecting personal and social data from women with breast cancer, readers are referred to Jeanne C. Quint, "The First Year After Mastectomy: The Patients and the Nurse Researchers," *Designs for Nurse-Patient Interaction*, Convention Clinical Sessions, Vol. 9, American Nurses Association (New York: American Nurses Association, 1964), pp. 5–12.

tients or provided information about incidents that had taken place at an earlier time. My intent was not so much to observe the students and teachers in action as it was to establish contacts with students while they were involved in assignments relevant to my interests. For example, I had several conversations with a student whose first patient assignment was a woman with advanced cancer. I continued to see this student at variable intervals during her three years in school. Fieldwork was vitally important during these early weeks because by being on the wards I was able to catch students while they were actively engaged in on-going assignments involving dying patients. I might note that neither the students nor the teachers classified some of the assignments which I found pertinent as necessarily related to death. On rare occasions, I also talked with patients.

My best sources for learning about students who had had critical incidents involving patients were other students. A conversation with one student frequently led to interviews with other members of her class. Teachers on the hospital wards also served as information resources by letting me know that certain assignments were in progress. As time passed, the teachers did not wait for me to appear on the wards but left messages, written or phoned, about incidents that they thought would be of value.

Although it was not difficult to hear about "death experiences" which the students were having or had had, making direct contact with these students was sometimes quite a different matter. In fact, some who had recently gone through traumatic personal experiences quite successfully evaded me when they knew that I wanted to talk with them. Also, other students and the teachers had a tendency to "protect" students from interviews with me if they thought the interview might cause the latter to become unduly upset. These behavior patterns were not unrelated to the problem being studied and also reflected the (middle-class) societal tendency to avoid conversations which might cause the person to lose control of his emotions. When I interviewed some students, they flatly stated that they would not have talked with me while certain incidents were in progress because they were too upset at the time.

Out of the many conversations with students and teachers came the development of working hypotheses which guided the collection of subsequent data. For example, the significance of first encounters with death as students was suspected and soon verified, but the relationships between assignment circumstances and the possible consequences for students (good, bad, or neutral results) were tentative until additional data could be gathered and analyzed. Analysis of early interviews suggested the relative importance of such assignment conditions as time in school, teacher expectations, teacher experience, assignment accountability, and high-risk wards.[8] Interest areas which appeared relevant to the students were identified and used as guides for later interviews. Data gathering had been in progress for about four months when contacts were made with the directors of the other four nursing schools to arrange for their participation in the study.

Interviews with Students

The students who were interviewed were not selected randomly. At the times when interviewing took place in each school, students were selected on the basis of established criteria such as year in school (first, second, or third) or assignment to a particular ward (medical, surgical, obstetrical, pediatrics, etc.). Because the study was focused on process, choice of interviewees on a random basis did not seem applicable, but might have been so had the schools been structured so that what happened to students followed a more rigorously consistent course. The selection of specific students by the school rather than by the investigator did not seem critically important or likely to produce a highly biased student viewpoint. This judgment was made on the as-

[8] High-risk wards were of two general kinds: those in which there was a high probability of students' having assignments to dying patients or direct encounters with death and those in which there was a high probability of personal involvement because of the patients' personal and/or social characteristics. The risk, in this instance, has reference only to students.

sumption that whoever chose the students would have limited knowledge about their actual experiences with dying patients. Some variation in experience was expected, but the wide variation reported by students in the same school was, in fact, a surprise to me. There was no reason to think that students were made available because they had had ideal experiences or presented the particular school in a highly positive way.

Most of the students participated in a single interview which averaged forty-five minutes. In two of the schools all the interviews were conducted in one day. In the other two schools, two sets of interviews were held three months apart. This pattern was used in order to talk with students shortly after they had completed their assigned weeks of psychiatric nursing experience. The interviews were conducted at the home school where room facilities were made available to the investigator. The interviews were recorded on tape and later transcribed in full.

The interviews were never highly structured and initially were quite general in approach, e.g., a student might be asked to tell about an encounter which she found particularly meaningful. (Commonly, meaningful encounters turned out to be recent experiences or those in which the students were actively involved at that point. Memories of more remote experiences seldom came out immediately, but emerged out of the process of talking together during the interview.) The later interviews were less generalized and focused specifically on areas about which questions had been raised by the preliminary analysis of data. In either case, the interviews were conducted to allow for the emergence of new categories of experience in addition to the verification, alteration, or disavowal of conjectured relationships among structural and experiential variables.

The interviews were conducted to maximize the opportunities for the students to talk freely about their encounters with death, their reactions to the experiences, and their feelings about themselves and about others. The students were told that whatever they said was confidential and would be used in such a way that they would not be identified personally. The establishment of trust was essential for the students knew I was also holding conversations with their teachers. The use of a tape recorder did not appear to inhibit free discussion by any of the interviewees. More commonly a student was hampered in expressing herself easily when the incident being discussed was one that precipitated intense feelings of a negative nature, e.g., personal negligence, intense sadness, or strong feelings of dislike for a patient. Some students apparently were disturbed at revealing themselves in a nonpositive light—to another person and to themselves as well. For others, the interviews served as emotional outlets for expressing thoughts and feelings that had sometimes been bottled up for a considerable period of time.

The substance of interviews with students who were seen on only one occasion depended somewhat on the reasons for having the particular conversation. When nothing was known in advance about the student's background, the initial problem was to learn whether or not the student had been present when a patient died or recalled a particularly meaningful assignment to a dying patient. The conversational content grew out of the actual experiences which the student described. The investigator's questions were designed to clarify such factors as the following: what took place; who was involved; what actions were taken by the student and by others; how she reacted; what events took place subsequently; what the experience meant to her. Sometimes the interview was sent in a new direction because the student's comments about a particular issue suggested the value of a shift in emphasis. In an interview with one senior student, for example, the conversation covered a wide range of topics, including the following.

1. A shock incident which took place during her junior year.
2. Feelings of depression provoked by patients who give up.
3. How she handled a conversation with a patient who tried to talk openly about dying.
4. The difficulties faced by the nurse during a nondisclosure assignment.

5. The wish to know herself if she were dying.
6. Other students serve as principal outlets when distressing assignments take place.
7. High variability in teachers as persons whom students can trust.
8. The sadness provoked by being with dying children.
9. The difficulties of working with families of dying children.
10. The differences between school assignments and hospital work assignments with respect to patient load and staff attitudes.

The nuances of personal reactions such as surprise, shock, or disillusionment showed most clearly in the interviews with first-year students—particularly when the conversations took place shortly after first encounters.

Some single interviews were arranged because the student's recent experiences were likely to provide new or missing data. Thus interviews were arranged to learn about traumatic incidents, challenging incidents, work assignments during the summer months, and many other events. Sometimes relatively short conversations were used to check out a particular idea, e.g., whether or not a student was choosing a particular course of action in an assignment which had been described by another person.

With some students a set of interviews was used. Sometimes the interviews took place over a period of several days and usually only one or two were recorded on tape. The technique of multiple interviews was used to collect data while a student was actively involved in an assignment to a patient who was dying. With other students the interviews were separated by a period of weeks or months and were done while the students were taking different nursing courses. A few students were seen at several points during the three years and shortly after they completed school and began to work in one of the local hospitals. Among the last group were a student who had been initiated into "death care" under relatively calm and supportive conditions, another who had learned how to talk with dying patients, and a third who had undergone rather traumatic experiences during the first year in school. Sequential interviews were also conducted with several graduate students whose major field of study was in medical-surgical nursing.

Interviews with Faculty

The interviews with faculty members were of several kinds, but all were unstructured in approach. Some were recorded on tape and were centered around the teacher's perspective on a particular incident in which a student was involved, as well as her own ideas about what was going on in a more general way among the students in the school. Some of the more formal interviews were focused primarily on the teacher's concerns and difficulties in working with students. In addition, a number of interviews were conducted with two or three teachers talking together as a group. Although most of the interviews with teachers were concerned with incidents in which students were intensely involved, a few were arranged because the teacher herself had undergone an intense or traumatic experience in the process of teaching.

A great many informal conversations were held on the wards, during coffee breaks, and during casual encounters in the hospital corridors. Some of these encounters were planned by me because I wanted to get the teacher's views on a particular incident. Some provided the chance to learn about assignments that I could not have discovered in any other way. Others were used to clarify the teacher's views on what was being taught about death as well as how the content was being presented. Not uncommonly, these conversations brought into sharp focus the discrepancy between a student's view of an issue or incident and the teacher's view of it. As was true in talking with the students, interviews with the teachers were conducted to maximize the opportunities for open and free discussion.

Other Data Sources

During the early phase of the study, an interview with the director of each school (or an assistant) provided an overview of the instructional program and its organization. The school bulletin was used as a resource for structural data which were later confirmed (or rejected) in a second interview with the same administrative representatives. Those two interviews were separated by a three-year time span, and the second conversation was also used to ascertain what changes had taken place in the school—including any curriculum revisions brought into being through participation in the study.

The data obtained from graduate students, including teachers who took summer school courses in cancer nursing, provided valuable comparative materials for understanding what took place during the process of becoming a nurse. Nursing textbooks and periodicals were analyzed to bring historical data to bear on the problem being studied and to provide a socio-historical framework within which to consider the findings provided by the primary data. A considerable amount of complementary data, which confirmed and supported the primary findings, was obtained through conversations with many practicing nurses during the data-gathering period.

Another set of data was provided through my experience as a teacher during this same period. As a guest lecturer (with time, I became a sort of expert on death), I had many opportunities to listen to students and teachers describe and discuss their experiences with dying patients and their reactions to them. In addition, I conducted special-study seminars for a few students—both undergraduate and graduate—who chose to study with me because of a special interest in dying patients or in patients with breast cancer. These students provided a rich resource of data about the process of identity change. They also helped me to clarify some ideas about the teacher's role in providing an environment in which the student could experiment with difficult interactions and could get help in understanding what she was doing. In the process of teaching, I was directly influencing what happened to these students and thus was altering the data which they were providing.

Analysis of the Data

The data were qualitative rather than quantitative. The analysis was essentially a search for patterns among the structural and experiential variables conceptualized during the first year, the stage of preliminary analysis.[9] From a perusal of fieldnotes and interviews came the development of the variables and working hypotheses which guided the on-going collection of data. Predictions were made and subjected to testing in subsequent interviews. The conceptualization of significant variables and the tentative formulation of relationships among them derived from an implicit coding of the data and were written into memos addressed to particular topics. Written during the first six months of the study, some early memos contained ideas that emerged as predominant themes when the data were later analyzed more systematically.[10]

During the second year a more systematic analysis and explicit coding of interview data began. Use of the data and the development of a conceptual framework were aided by frequent conferences with one or both of my colleagues. The data were scrutinized carefully for similarities and differences in the two critical problems, conversations with dying patients and encounters with death. Analytic memos were written to delineate in precise terms the many variations in these critical experiences, and to clarify the structural conditions that maximized or minimized the chances of certain results. Key properties of the as-

[9] Structural variables are social conditions and personal characteristics that serve to define the context of an experience. Assignment length and time in school are examples of structural variables. Experiential variables are the responses made to an experience. Expectations, reactions, verbal and non-verbal strategies are examples of experiential variables.

[10] The early memos included these topics: rotation system and student encounters with death; first-time encounters, anticipated and not anticipated; some consequences of using a teaching hospital for student assignments; encounters with death—the importance of negligence; faculty as models for students; student accountability—to whom, for what, and how; conditions that maximize trauma for the student.

signment context were identified, and their effects on student experience were sharpened. Some statements from a memo on accountability can serve to illustrate the point.

Now, students are held accountable for certain assigned events, but they constantly encounter unassigned events, the latter running the gamut from "nice" to "awful." Conversations with students indicate the *salience of unassigned events* in student nurse work experience.

As the analysis continued, the relative importance of other properties was brought into focus—thus, the category of student ignorance became a powerful explanatory variable. As a final step, I examined the developmental effects of critical encounters with dying patients and with death as they were reflected in the behaviors of students at different points in the process of becoming nurses, and compared these behaviors with the actions and attitudes of nurses already in practice.

The Investigator: Some Problems and Stresses

To begin with, my participation in the study was not accidental. It happened because some intense personal experiences with death produced changes in me and in my view of living. In fact, an invitation to join the project was extended in part because I was a nurse who was relatively comfortable in talking with people about the process of dying. As a nurse and as a former teacher of nurses, I brought to the project many attitudes and conceptions about patients and about nurse students, as well as some deep concerns about the unpleasant things I had seen happen to both groups in the hospital. In having this information, the reader is in a better position to judge and to question what I have written.

As a nurse now assuming the role of sociologist, I was moving back into an old familiar setting with a "new set of eyes." Shortly after I began talking with students, however, I became aware that the experience was having an interesting effect. I began to recall many different death incidents in which I had been involved as a nurse—and some of these were not without a twinge of emotional distress. For the first time in years, I thought about my own experiences as a student. In a memo written during the first month, I had commented,

> One thing that stands out in my mind about training was the lack of sympathy and understanding which students were shown by supervisors and head nurses. You learned early that you were not to make mistakes—and you learned to stay out of the way of the head nurse. I can remember hiding in the utility room when Miss L. came down the hall.

> You learned not to talk back. I learned that the hard way. I can remember this nurse in the operating room. I had a headache that morning and talked back to her. I can remember her standing by my shoulder—I was scrubbed in on some kind of surgery. She stood there and told me off in front of the doctors and everyone. How I hated that one. And I still carry strong feelings of resentment toward people who treat one with such contempt.

The process of talking with students about their experiences (as students) was causing me to relive some of my own.

Perhaps because of my early experiences, it was easier for me to identify (possibly at times to overidentify) with the students than with the teachers—even though I had also been a teacher. For whatever reasons, I was less sympathetic and understanding of the teachers' problems than of the students' until a conference with the project director brought this partisan viewpoint sharply into focus. I had a tendency to be concerned about the individual who, in my judgment, held the position of underdog. My participation on a project about dying patients and hospitals is in itself an expression of such concern.

In the role of interviewer, I introduced myself as a nurse and made no secret of my prior work experience in schools of nursing. Because I was asking individuals to talk openly and frankly about personally meaningful (sometimes highly dramatic or deeply poignant) experiences, I viewed my role as confidante very seriously. Thus I took pains not to discuss the content of the interviews except during work sessions with my colleagues on the project.

The interviews themselves were surprisingly easy to conduct—even on occasions when the interviewees were emotionally disturbed. There were some exceptions, and I found that I became uncomfortable while talking with students or teachers who held themselves in tight emotional control. When this reaction occurred in me, it was often accompanied by a feeling that the other person really did not want to be interviewed and to talk about potentially upsetting materials. My greatest upset came following an interview with a nurse who had discovered the body of a patient who had committed suicide. I was disturbed because I thought the interviewee herself was ready to fall apart emotionally, with the interview serving as a triggering mechanism. In that event, I would be reprimanded for causing a scene. In a very personal way, I was reminded that nurses (or, at least, I as a nurse) are supposed to prevent scenes, not to provoke them.[11] This insight, as well as others, came to conscious awareness through my discussions with the project director and were useful in interpreting some of the data.

During the second year of the study, the students' view of my role came to light. From a student who accidentally spilled the beans, I learned that among the undergraduate students on campus I was known as the "death nurse." One student cogently stated the proposition, "What kind of kook would want to talk about death all the time?" I interviewed another student a year after she had graduated and heard these statements, "I think basically I didn't want to talk to you because you were the symbol of the death lady. I just didn't really want to talk to you because you were the huge symbol of massive bad illness." Her comments only confirmed what I had already learned from personal experience. Dying is a topic which many people do not want to discuss—even in the abstract. When I mentioned my work to friends or acquaintances, the usual reaction was "how depressing" or "how can you stand it."

11 See Barney G. Glaser and Anselm L. Strauss, *Awareness of Dying* (Chicago: Aldine, 1965), pp. 158–161, for a discussion of status-forcing scenes used by nurses and family members to achieve certain goals.

My final comments have to do with what was for me the most difficult problem, that of being a sociologist. My research training had been eclectic rather than specialized, and it had been super-imposed on a practitioner perspective acquired through some twenty years of experience. My views of the world and my modes of thinking were markedly different from those of my colleagues. As sociologists, they used a language which at first I did not understand. Thus I frequently found myself in a position of asking for interpretation. For about six months, I was acutely aware of feelings of inadequacy and inferiority. In retrospect, I cannot say at what point the change began, but one day the language of categories and theories no longer posed a threat. The analytic process, however, was never easy. The interpretations and ideas in the book are subject to these limitations in my research training and experience. In knowing my background, the reader can better judge the merits of what I have written.

Appendix B | Some
Assignment
Policies

SCHOOLS	A			B			C			D			E		
YEARS	1	2	3	1	2	3	1	2	3	1	2	3	1	2	3
Hours of clinical practice per week *	8	18	18–24	24	24–40	24–40	15	20–25	25	10	24	24	24	24–40	24–40
Use of evenings		x			x	x			x			x	x	x	x
Use of nights						x			x			x			x
Use of weekends					x	x			x				x	x	x
Weeks of vacation per year	18	18	18	4	4	4	10	10	10	8	8	8	4	4	4
Hospital work for pay permitted	x	x	x		x	x		x	x		x	x		x	x
Affiliated experience Other Hospitals	x				x	x		x	x			x		x	x
Other community agencies			x		x	x		x			x				x

Administrative Relationships: School A, university

Schools B and D, hospital affiliation, school a separate division

Schools C and E, hospital affiliation, school and nursing service combined

* All schools were on a semester basis except School E which used the quarter system. During the first semester of the first year, all schools utilized approximately the same numbers of hours for clinical practice each week: from 3 to 6. During the second semester (or third quarter) of the first year, schools showed greater variation in the amount of time devoted to clinical practice, as is indicated above.

273

Index

A

of conversations, 112
of dying patients, 176
of interactions, 234
of negligent performance, 38
patterns of, 176
of pediatrics, 178
of personal contact, 75
of personal involvement, 133

Awareness, advance, 151
closed, 82n, 90
shift of, 95
of dying, 87, 100, 112
lack of. *See* Lack
mutual pretense, 82n, 91
open, 82n, 95, 156
suspected, 82n, 90

B

Babies. *See* Children
Baccalaureate nursing program, 16, 17, 19, 27, 29–30, 36n, 38–39, 54–55, 175, 255. *See also* School, of nursing graduate of, 60
"Back stopping," 69, 76, 242
Basic educational programs, 199. *See also* Nursing curricula; Nursing education
Basic students, 104, 167–83. *See also* Student nurse(s)
Beginning students. *See* Student nurse(s), first-year
Behavior, in bereavement, 4, 6–7, 58
bizarre, 243
collective, 21
inappropriate, 150, 157–58
irreverent, 123
of patient. *See* Patient
pattern, 260
professional, 64, 166
responsible, 23–24, 47
"right," 21n
science of, instruction in, 256

content, 235, 242
of sick adults, 166
stereotypical, 115n
Beliefs, 10, 37, 118, 228, 236
about death, 2, 227
Bereaved person, 6–7, 7n, 111, 111n, 151–52. *See also* Bereavement; Feelings, of loss; Grief; Mourning
Bereavement, 4, 6–7, 7n, 14, 58, 115n. *See also* Bereaved person; Feelings, of loss; Grief; Mourning
Biological science, instruction in, 256
Biopsy, 97. *See also* Cancer
Birth, 1n–2n, 164–65
and deformed baby, 165
Blame, 110, 141, 143, 149, 187, 222, 231. *See also* Feelings, of guilt; Negligence, concerns about
Blunders, 204, 207
Body. *See* Corpse
Breast, biopsy, 97
cancer, 259n. *See also* Cancer

C

Chaplain, 108, 198, 215. *See also* Clergymen; Minister; Priest
Characteristics, esteemed, 101
  highly valued, 44, 118
  social, 101
Chart, of patient, 105
Children, 118, 131, 132
  with fatal illnesses, 102–103, 106–108, 178, 242–43
  premature, 128
Chore. *See* Work
Classroom, discussion in, 58, 67–68, 70–71, 80, 134, 195, 237
  use to ventilate, 160
Clergymen, 12n, 21, 108, 109, 160, 213–16, 250. *See also* Chaplain; Minister; Priest
Clinical nursing, 16
Clinical practice, 36n, 83
  fields, 24
Clinical setting, 58–59. *See also* Hospital, locale
Clinical supervision, 26, 35. *See also* Supervision, of student performance
Clinical teaching. *See* Teaching, in clinical setting
Clue, 89, 90, 96
Colleague, 100, 270, 271
Collegiate nursing program. *See* Baccalaureate nursing program
Colostomy, 57
Comfort, 197, 202–204. *See also* Care, and comfort
  painless, 173–74
  physical, 57, 210, 221
Commendation, from staff, 154
Comment. *See also* Conversation
  innocent, 94

nonspecific, 105
Commonsense judgments, 79, 109, 112, 144
Communication, 231–34, 241
  channels, 116
  difficulties, 53
  lack of, 232
  open, 197
  with patients, 79n
  with physicians, 51, 189
  problems, 233
  skills, 17, 29–30, 39
Community hospital. *See* Hospital, community
Companionship, 202
Compensations, for dying patients, 202
  for helpless feelings, 108, 112
Competence, lack of, 135–37, 182. *See also* Inadequacy
Composure, 44
  management of, 173–74
  strategy, 34n
Conceptualization, 267
Concern, for classmate, 136
  about pain, 94
  of primary, 107
  teacher, 49, 66–69
  of students, 134–39. *See also* Negligence, concerns; Student nurse(s), perspective of
  about what to say, 80
Condition(s), contributive to traumatic incidents, 34
  for difficult talk, 98
  of dual responsibility, 48
  structural, 255
Conference, 267
  individual, 39, 41, 54, 195, 255–56

D

E

F

Blame; Negligence, concerns about
of helplessness. *See* Helplessness
of loss, 101, 115n, 118, 151–52. *See also* Bereavement; Grief; Mourning
negative, 149, 263
of negligence. *See* Blame; Negligence, concerns about
positive, 149
of sadness. *See* Grief; Sadness; Tragedy
of social loss, 108
Fieldwork, 4, 258–61. *See also* Research
data, 253, 253n, 254
notes, 258, 267
Fieldworker, 258
First-time experiences, of students. *See* Student nurse(s)
First-year students. *See* Student nurses, first-year
Flexibility, of approach, 4, 257
Forewarning, 78, 133
Fragmentation, 50–51
Frame of reference, 7
Framework, sociohistorical, 266
stereotyped, 56
Frustration, 60, 68, 71, 98, 115, 197, 241
Fundamentals of nursing, 31–32, 57, 255–56
Funeral, 2

G

"Generalist," 55
Genitals, handling of, 251
Geriatrics, 14
Gerontology, 58
Goal, 22, 42, 107
Go-between, 233
Grades, 37
Graduate nursing program, 4, 189, 244, 250
students in, 9, 41, 69, 104, 189–96, 197, 212, 265
Gratification, 9, 146, 184, 196–97
Grief, 6, 7n, 14, 35, 58, 68, 111, 115, 116, 118, 120n, 132, 145, 151–53, 218, 248–49.
See also Bereavement; Feelings, of loss; Mourning; Sadness; Tragedy
Group conference, 41
Guest lecturer, 266
Guidance, 67, 110–11, 160, 243. *See also* Direction
little or no, 42
to nursing staff, 246
of training experience, 243
Guidelines, 45, 58, 68, 79, 196. *See also* Rules
few, 144, 186
Guilt feelings. *See* Blame; Feelings, of guilt; Negligence, concerns about

H

J

K

L

M

Nursing curricula; Undergraduate nursing program
Nursing publications, 14. *See also* Journals, nursing; Textbooks, nursing
Nursing school. *See* School, of nursing

Nursing service, 15, 174n, 246, 256
Nursing staff, 193, 196–97. *See also* Hospital, employees
Nursing standards. *See* Standards
Nursing students. *See* Student nurse(s)

O

Obligations, social, 7
Observation, 83–84
  for changes, 20, 23
  skills required for, 255
Observer, 42, 114
Occupational therapy, 81
Operating room, 117, 131, 157
Operation. *See* Surgery
Opportunities, to cry, 206
  to deal with feelings about death, 175
  to encounter death, 28, 32
  to grieve, 217–18

  to talk, 160–61, 205
Orderly, 123, 125
Organization, of course work, 19–20
  of school, 19, 24–36, 73–76, 243–44, 255
Orientation, toward death. *See* Death
  to nursing practice. *See* Nursing practice
  sociological, 257
  theoretical, 4–7
Outsider, 53, 117, 120, 131, 193

P

Pacemaker, 213
Pain, 135, 146–47, 174, 210, 212–14, 251,
  agony of, 212–14
  medication for, 23, 224
  relief of, 20, 22, 224
  worry about, 99
Participation, in class, 37
  by physicians, 51

Patient, anger of, 118, 196
  antagonistic, 220
  assignment to, 24, 29–32, 38, 41, 60, 95, 172. *See also* Assignment
  conditions, 42–47
  difficult, 242
  first, 139–40
  hazardous aspects, 240

R

S

of loss; Grief; Mourning;
Tragedy
Safety, discrimination for, 105
of patients, 25, 64
Sanctions, social, 7
Satisfaction, 9, 10, 196
Scapegoat, 44
Scene, 269, 269n
School, 5–6, 27, 54
assignment by, 18, 27, 36–37,
47, 114, 202, 238–41. *See
also* Assignment; Patient, assignment to
bulletin, 266
environment of, 241. *See also*
environment
of nursing, 2, 4, 7, 10, 16–18,
54–55, 69, 73, 75–76, 247–
48, 254. *See also* Baccalaureate nursing program;
Hospital nursing school
objectives of, 24
requirements of, 37
Search, for patterns, 267
for support, 69, 71, 109–110
Second World War, 15, 50
Sedation, 23. *See also* Medications
loose orders for, 187
Selection, of patients, 32, 34–35,
54, 59, 65
of students, 261
Self, accusation of, 141, 149
appraisal of, 5
control of, 44. *See also* Control
evaluation of negligence by,
190. *See also* Accusation of
negligence; Blame; Negli-
gence, concerns about
Semester, first, 32
Seminar, 72, 192

special-study, 266
Senior student. *See* Student
nurse(s), senior
Sensitivity, 30, 39, 43, 85, 129
psychological, 213
Separation, between medicine and
nursing education, 51–52
of nursing education and nursing service, 51–53
Septicemia, 122
Shock, 121, 123–24, 128. *See also*
Impact; Involvement
emotional, 251
reaction to, 149, 156–58, 251
response to, 150
sensory, 117
Sign, observable, 107
warning, 107
Significance, of nurse-patient conversation, 93
psychological, 6
special, 120
Situation, impossible, 66
stress, 256–57
threatening, 166
traumatic, 131
Skill, 136
specialized, 13
Sleep, disturbance in, 157, 161
Social loss. *See* Loss, social
Social science, 242
literature of, 12
Social scientist, 1, 7n. *See also*
Sociologist
Social worker, 66, 70, 72, 108
Socialization, 5n, 78n, 162
agency for, 2, 4. *See also* School
process of, 5, 36, 78
techniques, 251

T

W

Y

DATE DUE